THE CONFIDENT HOME COOK

Dinner For One

(One Pan, One Plate, One Happy Belly)

Healthy Cooking for One Person: Quick, Fun, and Easy Meals with Big Taste and No Waste

Kerstin Decook

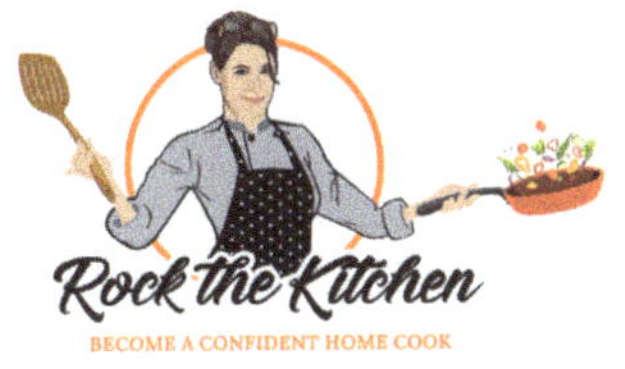

THE CONFIDENT HOME COOK

Dinner For One

(One Pan, One Plate, One Happy Belly)

Kerstin Decook

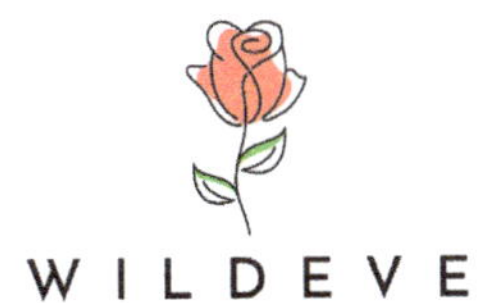

WILDEVE

THE CONFIDENT HOME COOK
Dinner For One (One Pan, One Plate, One Happy Belly)

All recommendations are made without guarantee on the part of the author or the publisher. The author and publisher disclaim any liability in connection with the use of the information contained in this book. This book is intended as a reference and guide only. The author and publisher are not responsible for any adverse effects or consequences resulting from the use of any recipes or instructions contained within. Always follow food safety guidelines and consult with a healthcare professional when necessary.

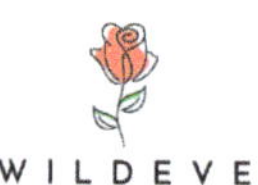

Paperback Edition ISBN: 979-8-9993526-4-4
Hardcover Edition ISBN: 979-8-9993526-5-1
Digital Edition ISBN: 979-8-9993526-3-7
LargePrint ISBN: 979-8-9993526-9-9

Library of Congress Control Number: 9798999352644

Cover illustration artist: Yvette Gilbert from the United Kingdom
Interior Illustration Artist: Lidia Nureeva from Kazakhstan
Book cover design and interior formatting: Van-garde Imagery, Inc.

Wildeve Press is an imprint of Vendela Publishing, LLC. Vendela Publishing is registered in the United States of America and other countries.

Contents

From Me to You . . . 9

Inspiring Praise from Beyond the Apron . . . 11

Praise from Real Home Cooks . . . 13

Introduction . . . 15

How to Rock This Book . . . 19

Welcome to Your Flavor Playground . . . 23

Kitchen Hacks to Simplify, Sassify, and Totally Upgrade Your Solo Game . . . 29

- Curry Me Home . . . 40
- Flat Out Fabulous . . . 42
- Balls of Glory . . . 44
- Egg-cellent for One . . . 46
- Pastably Perfect Mini Bake . . . 48
- Shrimply Divine . . . 50
- Get Your Wrap Together . . . 52
- Taco Me Later . . . 54
- Let's Have a Pep Talk . . . 56
- Shroom for One . . . 58

Eggs in a Hot Tub 60
Bangkok in a Pan 62
Mac My Day. 64
Bake It Till You Make It 66
Veggies Gone Wild 68
Egg-cuse Me, Dinner? 70
Frittata Me Not 72
Umami in a Hurry 74
Holy Frijole 76
Wrap Me Baby One More Time 78
Crust Me, It's Good 80
Flavor Jacuzzi 82
Tossed and Sauced 84
Soba Noodle Alla You 86
Lemony Snickerdish. 88
Fire & Lime Affair 90
Comfort in a Cup (or Bowl) 92
Tabbouleh, Your Way 94
In a Pickle (and Loving It) 96
Bowl'd & Boujee (Fancy, That Is!) 98
Pasta La Vista, Boring 100
Ricotta Be Kidding Me 102
Queso Amor 104

Fry Me to the Moon. 106

Board Out Of My Mind 108

Solutions for When You'd Rather Snack Than Sauté 111

Bonus: Sauce It, Stir It, Drizzle It 113

Peanut Sauce, Please!. 114

Pesto Party for One 115

So Low Hummus 116

Sriracha Mayo (or Yogurt) 117

Chipotle Mayo (or Yogurt) 118

Quick Drizzles & Dollops 119

The End? Nah. Just the Delicious Beginning. 121

A Little Flavor Favor. 122

The Menu: Dished Out 125

The Menu: Served by Style 127

Bake Squad 127

Egg-citing Eats 127

Fresh Fix 127

Grainfully Delicious 128

Noodling Around 128

Slurp Worthy 128

Snack-Cuterie 129

Stir Crazy 129

Toastally Topped 129
Wrap Stars 129
Bonus: Sauce It, Stir It, Drizzle It 131
About the Author 132

From Me to You

Before we dive into one-pan magic, flavor bombs, and solo-sized wins, let me start by saying: I'm so glad you picked up this book.

Whether you're here because cooking for one feels a little *meh*, or you're tired of eating snacks over the sink — welcome. You're in the right place.

Maybe you've lost the motivation to make a "real" meal just for yourself. Maybe you're tired of recipes built for four when you're flying solo. Or maybe you simply want dinner to feel like *something* again — not another mindless chore at the end of the day.

Wherever you're starting from, I see you — and I promise, we're about to make solo cooking way more delicious (and a heck of a lot more fun).

This book was born from a conversation with a friend who said, "Cool, cool — you're writing a book about making salad dressings from scratch, but how about a book for all of us flying solo in the kitchen?"

He knows his way around a stove, but when it's just him, inspiration flatlines. I heard that and thought: *challenge accepted.*

And right there — the title was born: *Dinner for One.* Because that conversation instantly reminded me of the iconic British sketch that's aired in Germany every New Year's Eve for decades. If you know, you know. It features Miss Sophie hosting her annual birthday dinner — for a group of friends who've all passed away. Her butler, James, heroically steps in to play every guest, delivering their toasts (and drinking every one of their drinks). As the night goes on, he gets increasingly sloshed, repeatedly trips over the tiger rug, and continues serving Miss Sophie as if it's all perfectly normal.

It's absurd, hilarious, and somehow timeless.

Now, I'm not saying your solo dinners need imaginary guests or a tipsy butler, but they *do* deserve a little more celebration. And a whole lot more flavor.

So, I rolled up my sleeves and whipped up thirty-five solo-friendly dishes. That's more than a month's worth of fast, flexible, flavorful, and — let's be honest — kinda fabulous meals.

But here's the kicker: with a few swaps and tweaks, those recipes turn into dozens more. We're talking enough combos to last three or four months — no repetition, no rut, just meals that match your vibe.

Because here's the thing: when cooking feels like a chore, nobody wants to do it. But when it's fun? When it feels like an act of joy instead of obligation? That's when the magic happens.

This is not your "perfect measurements and rigid rules" kind of cookbook. It's more like me popping into your kitchen in comfy pants, handing you a wooden spoon, and saying, "Let's play."

Cooking for yourself is a choice. You can either dread it or turn it into a delicious little rebellion. I vote for the latter.

So, let's do this. Let's turn *Dinner for One* into a whole vibe. A happy-belly, confidence-boosting, flavor-packed adventure.

Shall we?

With flavor love,

Kerstin

Inspiring Praise from Beyond the Apron

"Kerstin Decook's *The Confident Home Cook: Dinner for One* isn't just another cookbook — it's a fresh, sassy, and inspiring guide to reclaiming joy in solo cooking. In a world where eating alone often means microwaved leftovers or lackluster takeout, Kerstin flips the script. She reminds us that cooking for one doesn't have to feel like a chore — it can be creative, fun, and even indulgent.

What sets this book apart is its refreshing attitude toward solo dining. Kerstin doesn't just share recipes — she builds confidence, one delicious, flexible dish at a time. Her no-fuss, flavorful approach paired with her signature humor makes this book feel like cooking alongside a witty friend who knows just how to spice things up.

If you've ever stared into your fridge wondering what to make, this book is your new kitchen wingwoman. Get ready to swap with confidence, plate with pride, and actually look forward to cooking for yourself."

— Randy Peyser, author of The Power of Miracle Thinking

"Want to simplify your life (and your cabinets)? *The Confident Home Cook: Dinner for One* is a sassy, uplifting companion that brings excitement and *yummy-ness* into your solo kitchen. Kerstin Decook's "Block Party" method encourages you to get creative with what you have on hand, turning mealtime into a flavorful, fun experience — with easy cleanup. Her vibrant voice and no-fuss style feel like a savvy friend standing at your side, guiding you through every dish.

You'll discover handy kitchen hacks that make solo cooking easier, reduce food waste, and help you use up leftover ingredients with flair. This book doesn't only teach you how to cook for one — it shows you how to make every meal a rewarding experience that's totally worth your time."

— Lana McAra, editor for AuthorOneStop

Kerstin Decook's meal-prep concept transforms cooking for one into a culinary adventure, regardless of one's skill level. In "The Confident Home Cook: Dinner for One", she swaps rigid measurements for a playful, intuitive approach to creating magic in the kitchen. All in the service of the most important diner: you.

As if anticipating the reader's self-doubt, Decook devotes the first third of her book to barrier-breaking tips on storage, shopping, and early prep. Her tone is pure encouragement—a "you can do this" pep talk from a trusted friend who also happens to be a leadership coach and award-winning writer. Clear, concise, and comprehensive, her instructions seem to speak directly to both the veteran cook and the timid solo cook. For busy professionals, college students, and newly single individuals, the frozen dinner may become a permanent memory.

— Laura Jo Brunson, Editor/Writer

Praise from Real Home Cooks

"What makes this book truly unique is its playful approach to cooking for one — helping you have fun in the kitchen while building confidence at the same time. The dishes don't just have fun names like *Bangkok in a Pan* or *Lemony Snickerdish* — they're actually fun to make, too, because you get options to use what you've got in the fridge or whatever needs using up. Kerstin gives you a framework for every dish, with plenty of flexibility to make it your own. It's a fresh, empowering approach that makes cooking something you actually look forward to. Five stars from this one-woman kitchen crew!"

— *Cherie Kukhahn*

Congratulations, Mrs. Decook! I love the innovative way you've tackled meal prep, storage, and cooking for us single guys — along with some beautiful-sounding recipes I can't wait to try! This book is a perfect pairing with "Dress to Impress", and I know I'll be using both in my kitchen.

— *Mike Hollan*

As someone who often eats solo (if you don't count the three dogs watching me), I'll admit I'm usually less than inspired to cook just for myself. It's not that I can't — I just end up digging through the freezer or daring myself to eat those leftovers before they turn into a science experiment.
When I got my hands on Kerstin's newest gem, I honestly felt like she wrote this book for me. The recipes I've tried so far have been quick, fun, and downright delicious.

Her tips and playful style give me just the right nudge to whip up healthy, flavorful meals that feel like a treat instead of a chore.

Dinner for One? Highly recommend — even if your dinner audience is just a pack of curious dogs like mine.

— Leon Ford

Introduction

If we haven't met yet — either through one of my cooking webinars, one of my books, or somewhere else in the wide world of flavor — allow me to introduce myself.

I'm Kerstin — a certified professional coach, author, speaker, and full-blown food enthusiast. But I didn't start out that way. I became all of those things by learning, doing, and letting myself grow (and burning a few dishes) along the way.

Back in the day, I cooked like many of us do: following recipes to the letter, winging it when I didn't know better, and turning out a few mystery meals without a clue why they were so good or what went sideways. And let's be honest — most nights, I cooked because I had to, not because I wanted to. It wasn't fun. It wasn't thrilling, and it sure wasn't creative. It was survival with a spatula — more chore than joy. Sound familiar?

That all changed when my husband and I launched an adventure charter business in the Pacific Northwest, and I suddenly found myself promoted (without warning) to Chef de Cuisine aboard a yacht. Fancy title, zero training. Cue panic.

Sure, I knew how to cook, mainly following recipes — but I wanted to do more than feed people. I wanted to wow them.

That moment kicked off my deep dive into the world of culinary arts. I didn't enroll to memorize recipes, I went to learn how to cook with confidence, creativity, and freedom. I trained in the U.S., Canada, and Europe to understand the *why* behind the *how* — learning techniques, flavor-building, and methods that transformed me from a recipe follower into someone who could create with ease and have a blast doing it. I learned to trust my taste buds, think like a chef, and turn everyday meals into little flavor odysseys — the kind where my husband rolls his eyes back and says, "Hey sweets… wow, this is good."

To be clear — he was perfectly fine with my cooking before. But now? He's asking what's for dinner before breakfast is even over, just so his taste buds can gear up for the ride. That's the magic of learning how to cook with curiosity, confidence, and a dash of play.

Fast forward to now, and the kitchen has become my happy place — my creative playground, flavor lab, and sometimes even my dance floor. I want to help you feel that, too.

Which brings us to this book

This book isn't here to boss you around or make you feel bad for skipping dinner or eating chips over the sink. It's here to help you reclaim dinner time. To ditch the stress. To stir up some fun. And to show you that cooking for one doesn't have to feel like a chore — it can be an act of self-care, joy, and straight-up delicious rebellion.

Now — before we jump straight to "Grab a pan and let's go"…

You might still be wondering:

> "But isn't it a lot of work just to cook for one?"
> "How do I not waste half the ingredients?"
> "What if I mess something up?"
> "How do I plan meals without overthinking it every day?"
> "What if I don't feel like chopping, shopping, or scrubbing a pile of dishes?"

Totally valid. I hear you. If you've ever defaulted to cereal, toast, or "snacks on a cutting board," you're definitely not alone.

These are the real hurdles that keep so many solo cooks stuck — and why this book was designed to meet you exactly where you are. You don't need more pressure. You need options. Flexibility. Flavor. And a few smart tricks that make the whole thing faster, simpler, and a whole lot more fun.

So, don't worry, friend — I've got you. Right after this intro, you'll find a section called **How to Rock This Book (and Your Solo Kitchen)**. That's where we'll unpack how to make this journey work for you: from figuring out what to eat, to getting in and out of the store (without buying 5 things that rot in the back of your fridge), to cooking with confidence and cleaning up with ease.

When you've got the right rhythm — and a little flavor love to back you up — cooking for one becomes less of a to-do... and way more of a treat.

Okay, now we're ready. Let's turn up the heat. Let's make it easy, exciting, and all about you.

How to Rock This Book

(and Your Solo Kitchen)

Before we dive into the fun stuff (spoiler: flavor bombs ahead), let's talk about the real stuff — the sneaky solo-cooking struggles that love to kill the vibe. We're calling them out, flipping the script, and showing them the door. Here are the usual suspects…

"What am I even supposed to cook?"

Planning solo dinners shouldn't feel like prepping for a board meeting. When your brain's fried and your fridge is a mystery box, the last thing you need is a complicated recipe with 17 steps and 3 specialty ingredients.

That's why this book keeps it chill — and flexible.

You'll get mix-and-match magic with zero stress:

Block Party Ingredients (your base), Power Players (pick your protein — or skip it!), Flavor Crew (herbs, spices & saucy extras), Wild Cards (the twist you didn't know you needed).

No rigid plans. No kitchen drama. Just a vibe-check and smart swaps to turn whatever's in your fridge into a dinner you'll actually want to eat.

No plan? No problem. Your next solo meal just became your chillest win of the day.

"Shopping for one is so annoying — everything comes in bulk!"

Preach. Who decided parsley had to come in a bouquet and tortillas in packs of 24?

That's why this book is packed with flexible, waste-busting tips to help you make the most of what's already in your fridge (yes, even that half-used bell pepper).

You'll get clever Wild Card ideas to roll today's leftovers into tomorrow's dinner without feeling like you're stuck on repeat, plus a whole section of hacks for storing, freezing, and keeping things fresh like a total pro.

Oh — and there's a tasty little bonus at the end that'll make solo cooking feel like the smart (and sassy) move it truly is.

No more bulk guilt. No more mystery mush. Just smarter shopping and dinners you'll actually look forward to.

"I hate chopping everything every night."

Same. Who has time to play sous-chef after a long day?

That's why *Plan-tastic Prep* is your new ride-or-die.

Spend a few chill minutes slicing, dicing, and feeling productive once a week — and skip the nightly chop-a-thon.

Think of it as future-you's love letter to tired-you.

Chop once. Win all week.

"Cleaning up for one? Total buzzkill."

That's why most of the meals in this book stick to one pan, one pot, or one trusty sheet pan — because who wants a mountain of dishes after a solo dinner victory? Not you. Not me. And definitely not your sponge.

Pre-cut parchment sheets? Total game changer. No scrubbing, no stuck-on mess — just a quick toss and you're done.

Sure, a few recipes might ask for a second pan (pasta and rice have their own drama, you know), but the mission stays the same: max flavor, minimum mess.

And here's a hot tip I live by: cook a batch of rice, quinoa, or pasta at the start of the week. That way, you're not boiling water every night like it's your part-time job. One pot, multiple wins — less cleanup, more couch time.

"I get halfway through cooking and realize I'm missing stuff..."
Ugh, been there — mid-sizzle panic is not the vibe.

That's why we're big on *Mise-teriously Efficient* — the setup hack that'll save your sanity (and your dinner).

A quick minute to gather your goods before the heat is on, and boom — you're cruising, not scrambling.

Because kitchen chaos, my friend, is optional.

"Honestly... I lose motivation when I'm cooking for one."
Totally get it. When it's just you, it's easy to think, "Eh, why bother?"

But that's exactly why this book exists.

The vibe here is simple: flexible meals, cheeky names, and just enough sass to make dinner feel like an act of joy — not obligation.

Let's turn *Dinner for One* into your favorite me-time adventure.

Welcome to Your Flavor Playground

Now that we've cleared the mental clutter (and maybe made you smile a little), let's talk about how this book actually works — and why it's not like the others.

You won't find any "Chicken with Mushroom Sauce" around here. Why? Because you might not like chicken. Or mushrooms. Or maybe you've got shrimp and spinach in the fridge instead. That's the beauty of this book — it gives you a recipe *framework*, not a flavor straitjacket. Each dish is built around fun, flexible building blocks that let *you* decide what goes on the plate.

You get to pick your ingredients, match them to your mood, and skip whatever doesn't vibe. The goal? To make solo cooking feel less like a chore and more like a creative jam session in your own kitchen.

Here's the layout you'll see again and again:

How It's Gonna Go Down – Your cooking method (Stovetop + Simmer, Oven + Roast… you get the idea)

Block Party (Ingredients) – Your flexible base: veggies, grains, and other building blocks

Call in Your Power Players – Protein options to match your mood (or what needs using up)

Assemble Your Flavor Crew – Herbs, spices, and saucy extras to bring the flavor

Here's the Game Plan – Easy step-by-step instructions to make it all come together

Play Your Wild Card – Tips, swaps, creative twists, and serving ideas to make it your own

This setup gives you structure *without* measuring-cup micromanagement. Unlike traditional cookbooks with rigid rules and one-size-fits-all portions — **you get options.**

We're not counting grams or weighing basil leaves.

You'll see real measurements in this book — tablespoons, teaspoons, cups — but they're guidelines, not rules carved in stone. **Each recipe is portioned for one satisfying meal,** but if you want more of one thing and less of another? Go for it. You do you.

You'll also see flexible phrases like a splash, a scoop, a drizzle, and a pinch. Here's the breakdown:

A splash = about 1–2 tablespoons

A scoop = around ¼ cup

A drizzle = just enough to coat or kiss the surface

A pinch = the amount you can grab between your thumb and forefinger (perfect for salt, spices, or sass)

When it comes to ingredients — especially in the **Veggies to Vibe With** section — treat everything like a suggestion, not a rulebook. Use what you love, what's in season, or whatever's looking a little too comfortable in your crisper drawer. Don't like something? Skip it. No stress.

One quick pro tip before you chop: You don't need a ruler in the kitchen, but you *do* want to cut your veggies into similar-size pieces. Why? Because **equal size = equal cook** — a lesson straight from culinary school that's saved many a dinner. It's the difference between "perfectly tender" and "why is this still crunchy?" Think of it like this: *same size, same cook, better bite.*

Not sure how to cut what? You don't need perfection — just aim for pieces that cook evenly and feel good in a bite. Here's a quick cheat sheet to get you started:

Spinach, kale, arugula – rough chopped

Tomatoes – diced or chunked

Bell peppers, zucchini, sweet potato – bite-sized pieces or small cubes

Corn, edamame, peas – already perfect as-is

Scallions, onions, shallots – sliced or finely chopped (your call!)

Mushrooms – sliced or quartered

Carrots, radishes, cucumber – thin half-moons, matchsticks or shredded

If a specific cut really matters — like thin slices for a stir-fry or cubes for roasting — you'll see a quick note in the recipe.

And what about your Power Players?

Just like your veggies, most proteins work best when cut into small, even pieces — especially for stovetop dishes like stir-fries or skillet tosses where you want quick, even cooking. Cubes, strips, or bite-sized chunks are ideal. But hey, if you'd rather sear a full fillet or roast a whole chicken thigh? Go for it — you're the boss of your own kitchen.

Hot tip: Bigger cuts (like a whole chicken breast or fish fillet) are great for oven bakes where slow, steady heat keeps things juicy. On the skillet? It's your call — cut it down or go big and bold. Trust your gut (and your cravings).

Flavor Crew Time!

Your Power Players (proteins) and Flavor Crew (seasonings like herbs and spices) come with plenty of wiggle room. These aren't rules — they're sparks. A flavor menu to inspire you, not box you in. Love a combo? Run with it. Not your vibe? Skip it.

The only Golden Rule? **Start small, then build.** Especially with bold flavors like garlic, hot sauce, spices, or dried herbs. You can always add more — but once it's in, it's in. So, go slow, taste as you go, adjust as you wish, and season to your satisfaction.

And hey, let's talk sauce.

Throughout this book, you'll see quick sauce suggestions — from spicy mayo to citrusy vinaigrettes — designed to bring your bowl, plate, or toast to life. You won't need to buy a bunch of fancy bottles that sit in the fridge door until they expire. Instead, you'll find a *Bonus Section* with some of my go-to homemade sauces: simple, small-batch, made with stuff you probably already have and *ready in literally minutes*.

No waste. No mystery ingredients. Just bold flavor in a few shakes, stirs, or swirls — made for real solo cooks, not restaurant kitchens.

Of course, you'll also see me call for classics like marinara or Alfredo here and there — I consider those your pantry pals, always ready to jump in and save dinner.

And here's the kicker:

Most meals take 30 minutes or less and use just one pan or a pot — sometimes both — or maybe a baking sheet. This isn't restaurant-style plating with three separate pots and a side of chaos. These are soulful, satisfying meals made fast — with easy cleanup that won't wreck your night. But hey, if you want to fry up a little steak or roast a fillet of fish on the side, I won't stop you. That's the whole point — *you're in charge*.

You can't mess this up. Really.

If something goes sideways — burnt edges, overcooked rice, sauce that tastes like confusion — don't panic. It happens to the best of us — me included. When things flop, I pause, take a breath, figure out what went off the rails, and make a note for next time. It's not failure — it's flavor research.

Progress over perfection, always. You're not trying to earn a Michelin star — you're trying to feed yourself something tasty. Every misstep gets you closer to cooking with confidence. Keep going. You've got this.

So, take a deep breath. This is supposed to be fun.

Your kitchen doesn't have to be perfect — it just has to be yours.

Psst... I've got something extra juicy waiting for you at the end of the book.

Bonus goodies like a 4-week solo meal plan, flexible shopping lists, and a pantry setup guide — all designed to make your solo kitchen life even smoother. *(Hint: it's my little thank-you for helping spread the word with a review.)*

Now that we've set the vibe, let's talk game-changers. The next section is packed with smart kitchen hacks that make solo cooking faster, easier, and stress-free. Let's go.

Kitchen Hacks to Simplify, Sassify, and Totally Upgrade Your Solo Game

Let's kick things off with a few gems that make cooking way easier — and way more fun. These aren't about fancy gadgets or complicated tricks. These are straight from real-life trial, error, and culinary-school ah-ha moments.

Deli-ciously Organized

The Storage Hack That Changed My Life

Want to simplify your life (and your cabinets)? Get yourself a stack of deli containers. Yep — the kind restaurants use. They come in 1-cup, 2-cup, and 4-cup sizes, double as measuring cups and storage, and best of all? One lid fits them all. No more playing match-the-lid with 27 sad plastic containers and still ending up with a mystery top that fits nothing.

They're perfect for prepping ingredients, stashing leftovers in the fridge, or freezing that second portion for a future you who doesn't feel like cooking. They stack like a dream, take up almost no space, and honestly? After I discovered them in culinary school, I donated my entire mismatched Tupperware drawer. Haven't looked back since.

Deli containers = chef-level organization with zero fuss. Trust me on this one. You can find them online if they aren't in your store.

Plan-tastic Prep

The Time-Saving Hack That's Got Your Back

Some nights, you want dinner *now.* Not after chopping three onions or waiting for rice to cook. These little time-saving tips have saved me from cereal-for-dinner more times than I can count:

Grain Game = Strong Cook a batch of rice, quinoa, or pasta at the beginning of the week and portion it into small deli containers. Or, grab a couple of ready-in-a-snap 90-second grain pouches — like Simply Nature's Quinoa & Brown Rice mix. It's all-natural, heats up in a flash, and tastes like you tried. Store leftovers in the fridge for a quick scoop in tomorrow's bowl. Just label and date your goodies - because nothing says "oops" like mystery goo with a side of fridge funk.

Chop Once, Cook Fast All Week Take 10–15 minutes one day to chop onions, mince garlic, and grate ginger. Store them in deli containers or zippered plastic bags. Want to level up even faster? Get a small food chopper (manual or electric, you choose) to blitz aromatics in seconds and clean up like a dream.

Pre-Cut Parchment Sheets = Kitchen Magic Buy pre-cut baking sheets. No measuring, no wrestling with the roll, no tearing weird edges. I keep mine stashed above the fridge, and they're my secret weapon for roasting, baking, and fast clean-up. One pan + parchment = no scrubbing. Yes, please.

Hot Tip (Without Heating the Whole House)

If you're wondering whether it's worth firing up the big oven just for one meal — I get it. That's where a small toaster oven or countertop convection oven can become your new kitchen MVP. It heats up fast, uses way less energy, and works beautifully for roasting veggies, baking small portions, or crisping up leftovers. No need to waste electricity when a little appliance can do big things. Go mini, get mighty, and cook with swagger.

Mise-teriously Efficient

The Setup Hack That *Will* Save Your Ass

Let's be real: nothing throws off your cooking groove like realizing halfway through that your garlic is burning... while you're still rummaging for the can opener. Or worse — discovering you're out of something *after* you've already started. Cue panic, burnt onions, and dinner derailed.

That's where the magic of ***mise en place*** comes in. Fancy French term, but don't let that scare you. It simply means "everything in its place." And trust me — ***mise en place*** **WILL save your ass.**

Before you get all hot and sauté-y:

Chop what needs choppin'.

Measure what needs measuring.

Grab your tools and ingredients.

And yes, re-read the game plan — even if you *think* you remember it.

This isn't about being a kitchen robot. It's about being **smooth, confident, and totally in control** once the heat is on.

Because when your garlic hits the pan, you don't want to be three steps behind with wet herbs and mystery spice jars. You want to be *ready to sizzle.*

And while you're rocking that smooth kitchen flow... here's another backstage gem from culinary school — a game-changing trick that spares you from the whole post-dinner chaos meltdown.

Lean? Clean!

"If you can lean, you can clean."

That little gem got drilled into us at culinary school — and they weren't kidding.

If you're just standing around waiting for something to simmer, you're missing a golden opportunity to wipe the counter, rinse that mixing bowl, or wrangle the spice parade back into the cabinet.

Clean as you go, and when dinner's ready, you're *not* staring down a mountain of dishes like it's Everest.

Half your kitchen will already be clean — Future you (and your sanity) will be doing a happy dance.

Half-ily Ever After

The Saver Hack That Rescues the Rest

Cooking for one often means using half an ingredient and wondering what to do with the rest. Here's how to stop wasting and start winning:

Citrus Saver 101

Used half a lemon or lime? Toss it cut-side up in a deli container with the lid on. It stays juicy, fragrant, and doesn't perfume your entire fridge. Bonus: squeeze a few into ice cube trays and freeze for instant citrus pop anytime.

Avocado SOS

Keep half an avocado from browning by leaving the pit in and brushing the cut surface with a little lemon juice. Wrap tightly in plastic wrap or place cut-side down in an airtight container. If it's already mashed, press a piece of plastic wrap directly onto the surface to minimize air exposure. Storing it in the refrigerator, ideally in the crisper drawer, will further extend its freshness.

Veggie Preservation Station

For halved veggies like bell peppers, onions, or tomatoes, wrap them tightly in plastic wrap or a reusable silicone cover. Better yet, pop them in one of your trusty deli containers — hint hint! This keeps them crisp, fresh, and ready when you are.

Freeze It Before You Lose It

Tomato paste, pesto, coconut milk, chopped herbs? Scoop into ice cube trays and freeze. Then pop the cubes into a deli container. Instant portion-sized flavor bombs, ready when you are.

Meat the Freezer Like a Pro

Big packs of ground beef, chicken, or pork aren't built for solo living — but you can be smarter than the package. As soon as you get home, portion your meat into dinner-sized servings that fit your appetite (think 4–6 oz if you're light, 8–10 oz if you're hungry-hungry).

Toss each portion into a freezer bag or a trusty deli container, label and date it, and stash it away. No more sad, gray meat getting fuzzy in the back of your fridge — just ready-to-roll protein when you need it.

Leftovers? Heck yes.

Most of these recipes make just enough for one with maybe a second portion (if you add more to the recipe) to stash for tomorrow depending on how hungry you are. Plan ahead and cook an extra meatball or grain bowl component while you're at it — that way tomorrow's dinner is halfway done before you even think about it.

Taste-fully Noted

The Flavor Journal Hack That Helps You Improve

This book isn't about following rules — it's about discovering what makes your meals taste amazing to YOU. That's where your Flavor Journal comes in. It's your space to jot down what you made, what you swapped, how it turned out, and what you'd try next time. You don't need to write essays — just quick notes that capture your flavor wins, creative twists, or delicious disasters (hey, we've all had a "what was I thinking?" moment).

You can start a separate journal, scribble right into these pages or grab the printable version in your bonus goodies (details at the end of the book) — whatever hits your fancy. Because the truth is: the more you reflect, the more you refine. And the more you refine, the more your taste game levels up. So grab a pen, stir in some self-discovery, and keep those flavor notes coming.

Spice-tacular Shifts

The Mini Mindset Hack That Keeps You Cooking

Let's get one thing straight: solo cooking isn't a sad consolation prize — it's a full-on celebration of you. But sometimes, when life gets busy or motivation dips, it's not your skillet that needs a shake-up — it's your mindset.

That's where these little spice-tacular shifts come in. Tiny tweaks in how you *think* about cooking for yourself can totally change how you *feel* about it.

No pressure, no perfection — just fresh ways to see your solo meals for what they really are: delicious acts of self-care, creativity, and a little rebellion against boring routines. (That's my coaching brain coming out to play — and believe me — it's ready to crank up the heat in your solo kitchen.)

Here's the secret sauce:

You're the Guest of Honor

If Miss Sophie can toast a room full of imaginary friends, you can absolutely roll out the red carpet for yourself. *Dinner for One* isn't second best — it's a celebration in your honor. And hey, if eating alone sometimes feels a little lonely? That's real, too — but every plate you serve yourself is proof that you're showing up for the person who matters most: you.

So, dust off the good plate, pour yourself a glass of something you love, and honor the most important guest at the table: your fabulous self.

Choosing to show up for yourself isn't just a nice idea — it's a declaration.

And trust me — you, my friend, deserve nothing less.

Music = Mood Magic

Turn up the tunes while you cook.

A kitchen dance break between sautéing and seasoning isn't optional — it's practically required.

It's impossible to stay stressed when you're grooving — and stirring is way more fun with a beat.

Treat It Like a Date (With Yourself)

Set the table. Light a candle. Plate your food like a boss — even if it's *just* you (especially if it's just you). You're not "eating alone" — you're celebrating yourself.

Mistakes = Flavor Research

Burnt garlic? Oversalted sauce? Welcome to the club.

Cooking oops moments aren't failures — they're flavor research for next time.

Take a note, laugh it off, and keep playing. (Chefs mess up, too — they just swear in French.)

Progress over perfection, always.

Smart Cooking Mindset: Make the Most of What You've Got

Cooking for one doesn't mean you have to worry about using up every single ingredient right away. The secret? Flexibility.

If you have half a bell pepper left after making *Bangkok in a Pan*, toss it into your next *Veggies Gone Wild* sheet pan meal. Leftover greens from *Bowl'd & Boujee*? Stir them into *Egg-cellent for One* for a quick, nutrient-packed frittata.

Think of your ingredients like building blocks.

Swap what you need. Use what you've got. Have fun while you're at it.

The Block Party method gives you permission to remix and match as you go. Cooking solo isn't rigid — it's your chance to create meals your way, reduce waste, and make it all feel a little more fun.

Bottom line?

When you shift your mindset, cooking for one stops feeling like a chore — and starts becoming a full-blown act of empowerment (and plate-licking joy). Change your thinking, and the flavor will follow.

And speaking of empowered thinking...

You might've noticed I skipped the fancy food glamour shots and went with watercolor illustrations instead. That's on purpose — because this book is about *real cooking* for *real people*, not magazine perfection. I chose watercolors to keep things fun, lighthearted, and flexible — to leave room for your own flair. Because *your dinner* doesn't need to look like *my dinner* to be absolutely delicious. This book is here to guide and inspire you, not intimidate you with pixel-perfect plates.

Still a little curious how some of these dishes come together? I've got you. Head to the ***Dinner for One Gallery*** on my website for a peek at the real-life meals I whipped up while testing these meal ideas. Scan the QR code below or visit **www.rockthekitchen.net/gallery**.

No filters, no fuss — just real meals made the Kerstin way.

Now that you're armed with hacks, mindset shifts, and a fresh new vibe… let's turn up the heat and rock your solo kitchen.

Quickstart Guide: One Pan, One Plate, Let's Go

1. Pick your vibe.

Craving cozy comfort? A bold stir-fry? Cheesy pasta? Flip through the recipes and follow your cravings.

2. Check your fridge.

Grab what you've got — those last few veggies, leftover chicken, or that half-used can of beans.

You don't need a full grocery run to make dinner happen.

3. Scan the recipe.

Each dish gives you options:

Block Party = your flexible base

Power Players = proteins (or not!)

Flavor Crew = herbs, spices, and sass

Game Plan = your steps

Wild Card = swaps, sauce tips, or creative twists

4. Make it yours.

The ingredients? They're suggestions, not rules.

Don't like something? Skip it.

Missing something? Swap it.

Not into the suggested protein? Go meatless — or add double cheese.

This is your dinner, your vibe, your rules.

5. Turn up the tunes and roll.
Cooking solo should feel like a celebration.

Fire up your playlist, pour a drink if you want, and enjoy the moment.

So what's calling your name — a bold bowl, a sizzling stir-fry, or a cheesy pasta night?

Whatever it is, grab your pan, crank up the heat, and make it yours.

Let's cook, solo superstar. You've got this.

Curry Me Home

A creamy, cozy stovetop curry that lets you follow your cravings. Bold, nourishing, and ready in about 30 minutes. Full of flavor, flexible by design, and so satisfying it practically hugs you back.

Prep Time: 10 min

Cook Time: 15–20 min

Total Time: 25–30 min

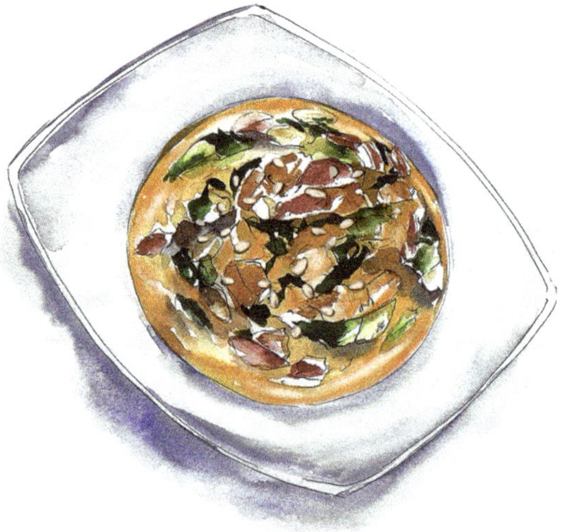

HOW IT'S GONNA GO DOWN

Stovetop Sauté + Simmer

BLOCK PARTY (INGREDIENTS)

For one hearty serving

1. **Veggies to vibe with (~1½ cups):** Bell pepper, sweet potato, potato, cauliflower, zucchini, spinach, corn or carrots
2. **Creamy element:** ~½ cup coconut milk (highly recommend), plain yogurt, or cashew cream
3. **Aromatics:** 1 garlic clove (minced), 1 tsp fresh ginger (minced), 1–2 tsp chopped onion, juice of ½ lime
4. **Optional grain base:** ½ cup cooked rice or quinoa

CALL IN YOUR POWER PLAYERS (~4–6 oz)

- Chicken breast or thighs (cubed)
- Shrimp
- Tofu (firm, cubed)
- Chickpeas (½ can, drained) or beans

No protein? No problem. *This curry is flavor-forward — the protein's just tagging along for the ride.*

ASSEMBLE YOUR FLAVOR CREW

- **Thai Team (Primary Pick):** curry paste (or powder), ginger, lime zest, basil, cilantro
- **Indian Team (For a twist):** turmeric, cumin, coriander, chili flakes
- **Drizzle Divas (Extra toppers):** toasted sesame oil, ghee, or olive oil

The Thai Team brings this dish together beautifully. Feeling adventurous? Try a remix with the Indian Team flavors.

HERE'S THE GAME PLAN – SIZZLE, SIMMER, SWOON

1. **Sauté aromatics** (except lime juice) in a splash of oil for 2–3 minutes.
2. **Add your protein** and sear if needed (skip this step if it's already cooked — like beans or pre-cooked chicken).
3. **Toss in the veggies** and stir things up.
4. **Add your flavor crew**, a pinch of salt, and the creamy element (~½ cup).
5. **Simmer** for 10–15 minutes until everything's cozy and tender. If using cooked grains, stir them in for the final few minutes so they warm through but don't go mushy.
6. **Finish** with a hit of citrus (lime juice!) and a sexy little drizzle from your Drizzle Divas lineup.

PLAY YOUR WILD CARD

- Use sweet potato or cauliflower for richness and body.
- Stir in a handful of spinach at the end for a pop of green.
- Craving a crunch? Rice crackers make a fun sidekick — but honestly, this curry stands proud all on its own.

Flat Out Fabulous

Crispy, cheesy, full of flavor — and yes, it steals the spotlight without stealing your time. With roasted veggies, bold proteins (if you're feelin' it), and melty cheese all piled onto one golden flatbread, this quick and customizable meal is everything dinner-for-one should be: easy, satisfying, and flat-out delicious.

Prep Time: 10 min

Cook Time: 20–25 min

Total Time: 30–35 min

HOW IT'S GONNA GO DOWN

Sheet Pan Roast + Broil

BLOCK PARTY (INGREDIENTS)

Makes one flat-out fabulous flatbread.

Base: 1 small flatbread, naan (GF if needed), flour tortilla, or your favorite bread

Veggies to vibe with (~1 cup): Mushrooms, cherry tomatoes, red onion, zucchini, bell pepper, leeks, arugula, spinach — or whatever's hiding in your fridge

Sauce (~2–3 tbsp): Pesto, hummus, marinara, or olive tapenade

Cheese (~¼ cup): Mozzarella, cheddar, feta, goat cheese, burrata, parmesan, or a dairy-free alternative

CALL IN YOUR POWER PLAYERS (~4–6 oz cooked)

- Grilled chicken
- Roasted chickpeas
- Tuna (drained and flaked) or smoked salmon
- Sausage (plant-based if you wish)
- Salami, ham, pepperoni or prosciutto

ASSEMBLE YOUR FLAVOR CREW

- **Italian:** oregano, basil, chili flakes
- **French:** herbes de Provence, thyme, oregano, basil, rosemary, cracked pepper
- **Latin:** cumin, chipotle, paprika, cilantro

HERE'S THE GAME PLAN – TOP IT, BAKE IT, FLAUNT IT

1. **Preheat oven** to 400°F (200°C).
2. **Toss chopped veggies** with olive oil, salt, pepper, and your favorite flavor crew. Roast for 15–20 minutes.
3. **Warm the flatbread** directly on the oven rack during the last 5 minutes.
4. **Spread sauce** on the warm flatbread, then pile on roasted veggies, protein, and cheese.
5. **Pop it back in the oven** and broil for 2-4 minutes, until golden and melty.
6. **Slice it up and enjoy** — no side dish required.

PLAY YOUR WILD CARD

- Top with fresh arugula or microgreens after baking.
- Drizzle with balsamic glaze or warm honey for flair.
- Optional extra: a crisp glass of white wine.

Balls of Glory

A handful of glorious meatballs made just for you (by you — ha!). Bold, juicy, and all kinds of flexible. Go meaty or plant-based, classic or spicy, paired with a rainbow of roasted veggies or tucked into toast — this cozy little dish delivers the flavor while the oven does the heavy lifting. Or keep it stovetop if you're feeling hands-on. Either way: pure glory.

Prep Time: 10–15 min

Cook Time: 20–25 min

Total Time: 30–35 min *(Most of it happens in the oven while you chill.)*

HOW IT'S GONNA GO DOWN

Oven Bake or Stovetop Sear + Simmer

BLOCK PARTY (INGREDIENTS)

Makes about 4–6 meatballs — enough for one glorious meal.

Pick your protein *(see Power Players below)*

1. **Veggies to vibe with (~1 cup total):** Bell peppers (any color), zucchini, mushrooms, red onion — anything roast-friendly and colorful
2. **Aromatics:** ~¼ cup finely chopped onion or shallot, 1–2 garlic cloves (minced), a pinch or two of chili flakes or smoked paprika (if you're feelin' spicy), a little chopped basil, and ~2 tbsp grated Parmesan *(optional)*
3. **Egg (optional):** 1 small egg or flax egg for binding

CALL IN YOUR POWER PLAYERS (~4–6 oz)

- Ground beef, turkey, pork, or chicken
- Lentils + grated mushrooms *(sautéed first)*
- Plant-based meat *(crumbled or shaped)*

ASSEMBLE YOUR FLAVOR CREW

- **Herby & Classic:** Basil, parsley, oregano
- **Spicy & Bold:** Chili flakes, smoked paprika, thyme
- **Earthy & Cozy:** Garlic, rosemary, mushroom powder or extra chopped mushrooms

HERE'S THE GAME PLAN – ROLL, LAYER, ROAST

1. **Preheat oven** to 425°F (220°C).
2. **In a bowl, mix** your protein, aromatics, egg (if using), and chosen flavor crew.
3. **Roll mixture** into 4–6 meatballs — roughly the size of a ping pong ball.
4. **Spread chopped veggies** onto a parchment-lined baking sheet.
5. **Nestle your meatballs** right on top of the veggies (one pan, no fuss).
6. **Drizzle everything** with olive oil, then sprinkle with salt, pepper, and a pinch of chili flakes or herbs if you like.
7. **Bake for 20–25 minutes**, until meatballs are cooked through and veggies are roasted and tender.
8. **Serve as-is or pile** them onto toast, grains, pasta — whatever you're feelin'.

PLAY YOUR WILD CARD

Want to sauce it up? Add during the last 5 minutes of baking or pour on when plating:

- **Roasted Red Pepper Sauce:** Blend jarred roasted peppers with garlic, tomato paste, olive oil, and a splash of vinegar.
- **Easy Marinara:** Grab your favorite jar. No shame, all yum.
- **Sweet & Tangy (German-ish):** Stir together ketchup, caramelized onion, a bit of olive oil, and a dash of vinegar or Worcestershire.
- **Prefer stovetop-only?** Sear the meatballs, toss in the veggies, and simmer everything together until tender and gloriously saucy.

Egg-cellent for One

A fluffy, flavor-loaded frittata made just for you. Raid the fridge, toss in your favorites, spice it your way, and bake (or finish on the stovetop) to golden, sizzling perfection. One pan, zero rules, and all the delicious payoff.

Prep Time: 5–10 min

Cook Time: 10–15 min

Total Time: 15–25 min

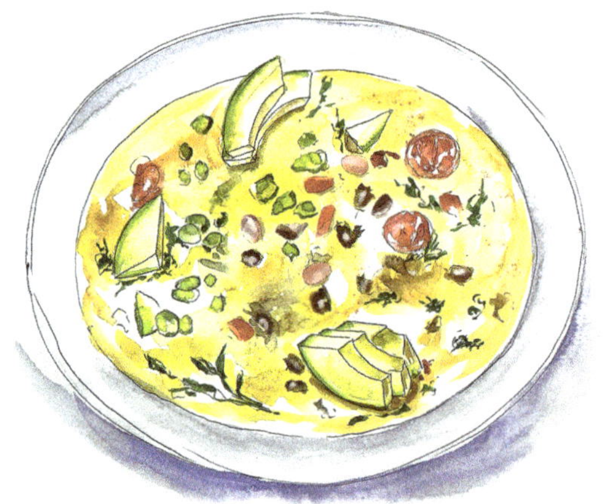

HOW IT'S GONNA GO DOWN

One-pan stovetop magic (or broiler finish)

BLOCK PARTY (INGREDIENTS)

Makes one generous solo portion.

1. **Eggs:** 2–3 large eggs
2. **Veggies to vibe with (~¾–1 cup total):** Bell peppers, onions, spinach, cherry tomatoes, zucchini, mushrooms
3. **Creamy bit (optional):** 1–2 tbsp milk, cream, or plain yogurt
4. **Cheese (~2 tbsp, optional):** Feta, cheddar, goat cheese — or your favorite dairy-free

CALL IN YOUR POWER PLAYERS (~2–4 oz)

- Diced ham or turkey
- Crumbled sausage (meat or plant-based)
- Smoked salmon
- Cooked lentils or black beans
- Or skip it — the eggs are holding court today

ASSEMBLE YOUR FLAVOR CREW

- **Italian:** Oregano, basil, garlic, Parmesan
- **Latin:** Cumin, paprika, chili flakes, cheddar
- **French:** Thyme, chives, gruyère or goat cheese

HERE'S THE GAME PLAN – STIR, POUR, SIZZLE

1. **Beat eggs** with salt, pepper, and your creamy add-in (if using).
2. **In a small skillet, sauté** your veggies and protein in a bit of oil until the veggies are tender and the protein is cooked through.
3. **Pour eggs over the top** and reduce heat to medium-low.
4. **Sprinkle with** your flavor crew (herbs and cheese).
5. **Cook uncovered** ~5–7 minutes until set.

PLAY YOUR WILD CARD

- Finish under the broiler for 2–3 minutes if you like that golden, slightly puffed top (just make sure your skillet is oven-safe and keep a close eye – it browns fast!).
- Want it grab-and-go? Let it cool, slice it, and pop it in a wrap or sandwich.
- Pair it with toast or salad if you're feelin' fancy — but it stands proud on its own.

Pastably Perfect Mini Bake

A cozy little pasta bake that's all yours — cheesy, saucy, and baked to golden, bubbly goodness. It's comfort food with just the right amount of indulgence, minus the mountain of leftovers. Yes, you'll use a pot, a pan, and a small baking dish (scandalous, I know). But trust me — totally worth it. Clean-up's easy: a quick rinse, a fast wipe, and parchment saves the day.

Prep Time: 10 min

Cook Time: 15–20 min

Total Time: 25–30 min

HOW IT'S GONNA GO DOWN

Stovetop Boil + Oven Bake (or toaster oven)

BLOCK PARTY (INGREDIENTS)

Just enough for one hungry belly.

1. **Pasta (~¾ cup dry / ~1½ cups cooked):** Penne, rotini, or elbows (GF if needed)
2. **Veggies to vibe with (~½ cup):** Spinach, mushrooms, zucchini, cherry tomatoes, bell pepper
3. **Sauce (~⅓ –½ cup):** Marinara, creamy tomato, pesto, or Alfredo
4. **Cheese (~¼ cup total):** Mozzarella, Parmesan, ricotta, or dairy-free shreds

CALL IN YOUR POWER PLAYERS (~4–6 oz)

- ➟ Cooked chicken or bacon
- ➟ Crumbled sausage (meat or plant-based)
- ➟ Lentils
- ➟ White beans
- ➟ Or skip it and go full cheese-mode

ASSEMBLE YOUR FLAVOR CREW

- **Italian:** Garlic powder, oregano, chili flakes, basil
- **Bold & Smoky:** Smoked paprika, cumin, onion powder
- **Fresh & Zesty:** Parsley, lemon zest, black pepper

HERE'S THE GAME PLAN – BOIL, MIX, BAKE

1. **Cook pasta** according to package directions. Drain and set aside.
2. **Sauté veggies** in a small pan with olive oil (~5 minutes).
3. **Add your protein** (if using), then stir in the sauce, your flavor crew, and half of the cheese. Mix in the cooked pasta and toss to combine.
4. **Transfer everything** to a small oven-safe dish (like a ramekin or mini casserole).
5. **Top with the remaining cheese and bake** at 375°F (190°C) for 10–15 minutes, until bubbly and golden.

PLAY YOUR WILD CARD

- No oven? Skip the bake — melt the cheese on the stovetop for a creamy skillet version.
- Want a crisp top without heating the oven? Pop it under the broiler or toaster oven for 3–5 minutes.
- This is the whole meal. Don't overthink it — just grab a fork and dig in.

Shrimply Divine

A Southern-style, spoon-to-belly solo dinner that's buttery, bold, and built to impress. Creamy grits or soft polenta set the stage while your shrimp, sausage, or sautéed veggies strut their stuff on top. It's rich, comforting, and—let's be real—shrimp-ly irresistible.

Prep Time: 10 min

Cook Time: 10–15 min

Total Time: 20–25 min

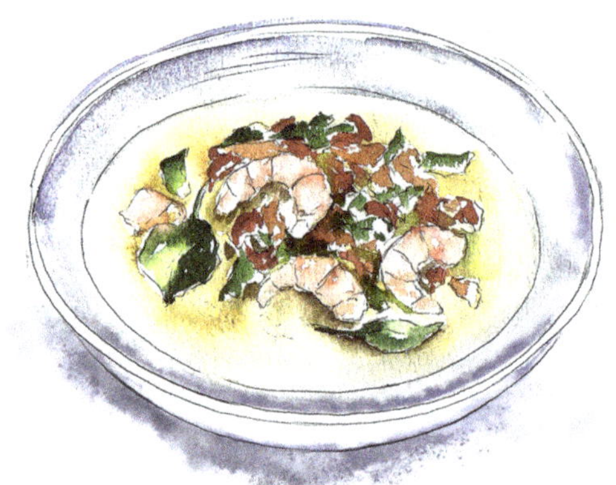

HOW IT'S GONNA GO DOWN

Stovetop Cook, Sauté + Simmer

BLOCK PARTY (INGREDIENTS)

Perfectly portioned for one full bowl of cozy.

1. **Grits or polenta (~¼ cup dry = ~1 cup cooked):** Quick-cooking or instant both work
2. **Liquid for cooking (~1 cup):** Water, broth, or a mix with milk for creaminess
3. **Veggies to vibe with (~½–¾ cup):** Spinach, tomato, bell pepper, corn, scallions, mushrooms
4. **Cheese (optional, ~2 tbsp):** Cheddar, Parmesan, or goat cheese

CALL IN YOUR POWER PLAYERS (~4–6 oz)

- ➟ Shrimp (peeled and deveined)
- ➟ Chicken sausage or andouille
- ➟ Bacon
- ➟ Crispy tofu
- ➟ *"Shrimp's the classic, but anything with a little sear will shine here."*

ASSEMBLE YOUR FLAVOR CREW

- **Cajun Kick:** Cajun seasoning, smoked paprika, thyme, garlic, chili flakes
- **Southern Comfort:** Cracked pepper, cumin, chili powder, butter + cheddar stirred into the grits
- **Tomato Twist:** Basil, oregano, garlic, cherry tomatoes sautéed with olive oil

HERE'S THE GAME PLAN – SIMMER, SIZZLE, SPOON IT UP

1. **Cook grits or polenta** according to package directions (simmer in water, broth, or milk mix). Stir in butter or cheese if using. Keep warm.
2. While that simmers, **sauté your protein** in a skillet until cooked through. Set aside.
3. In the same skillet, **add your veggies** and flavor crew. Sauté for 5–7 minutes until golden and tender, then return the protein to warm through.
4. **Spoon the creamy base** into a bowl and top with your sizzling skillet mix.
5. **Finish with fresh herbs**, a dash of hot sauce, or a drizzle of olive oil.

PLAY YOUR WILD CARD

- Want it saucy? Add a splash of broth or lemon juice at the end to make a quick glaze.
- Spice level's up to you — go bold if you love heat, or keep it mellow and buttery.
- Bonus move: Stir in a spoonful of pesto or chimichurri for a herby upgrade.

Get Your Wrap Together

Light, crisp, and packed with flavor — these lettuce wraps are your go-to when you want something fresh, fun, and fast. Use whatever you've got in the fridge and wrap your way to satisfaction. No fuss, just fabulous.

Prep Time: 10–15 min

Cook Time: 0–5 min (optional)

Total Time: 10–20 min

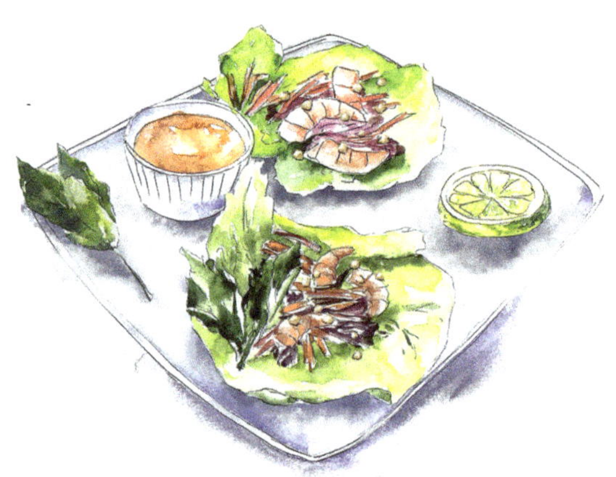

HOW IT'S GONNA GO DOWN

No-Cook or Quick Sauté

BLOCK PARTY (INGREDIENTS)

Build 2–3 wraps for one hungry human.

1. **Wrap base:** Butter lettuce, romaine, collard greens, or cabbage leaves
2. **Veggies to vibe with (~½–¾ cup crunchy fillers):** Shredded carrots, bell pepper, cucumber, cabbage, scallions
3. **Sauce (~2–3 tbsp):** Peanut sauce, sriracha mayo, yogurt-tahini, simple vinaigrette, or soy-ginger drizzle
4. **Optional toppings:** Crushed peanuts, sesame seeds, lime juice, chopped herbs

CALL IN YOUR POWER PLAYERS (~4–6 oz)

- ➡ Shredded rotisserie chicken
- ➡ Canned tuna or chicken (drained)
- ➡ Shrimp or tofu
- ➡ Tempeh, white beans, or lentils
- ➡ Leftover ground meat or plant-based crumbles

"Leftovers? Fabulous. Fresh? Even better. These wraps love whatever you've got."

ASSEMBLE YOUR FLAVOR CREW

- **Asian-Inspired:** Ginger, garlic, soy sauce, sesame oil, chili flakes
  Great with: tofu, chicken, peanut sauce
- **Latin Flair:** Cumin, paprika, lime juice, cilantro
  Great with: beans or ground meat, avocado
- **Mediterranean Fresh:** Lemon zest, dill, oregano, feta or tzatziki
  Great with: lentils, chicken, yogurt drizzle

HERE'S THE GAME PLAN – FILL, WRAP, CRUNCH

1. **If sautéing protein or veggies, start here:** Heat a little oil in a skillet and sauté your protein and/or veggies along with herbs or spices from your flavor crew. Cook until golden and done (about 3–5 minutes). Let cool slightly — you don't want a soggy wrap situation.
2. **Lay out your lettuce** leaves like taco shells on a plate.
3. **Pile in the crunchy stuff** — chopped veggies & your protein (warm or cold — your call).
4. **Drizzle or dollop** with your sauce of choice.
5. **Sprinkle with toppings** — a little crunch or creamy touch takes it next level.
6. **Wrap and crunch** — or eat open-faced with a fork if that's your vibe.

PLAY YOUR WILD CARD

- Not a lettuce fan? Use a tortilla or go grain-bowl style over quinoa or rice.
- Short on time? Keep it no-cook with canned beans, rotisserie chicken, or tofu straight from the fridge.
- Sauce swap? Try spicy mayo, tangy vinaigrette, creamy tahini — or all three. Who's judging?

Taco Me Later

A flavor-packed taco bowl that skips the tortilla (if you want) — but definitely not the attitude. Bowl it up, wrap it up, or pile it high. However you roll, it's fresh, fast, fiesta-flavored, and fully customizable.

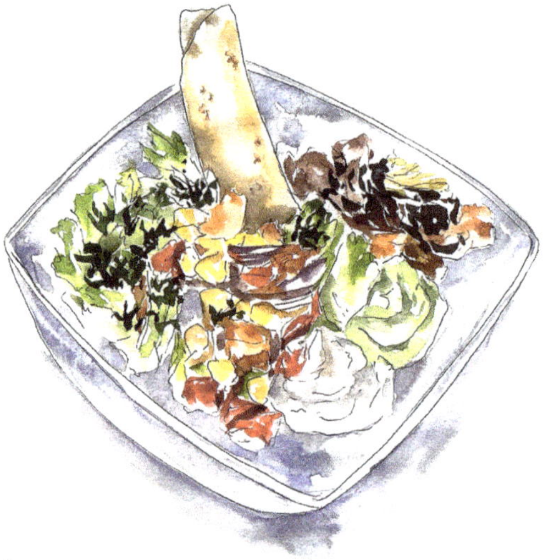

Prep Time: 10–15 min

Cook Time: 5–10 min (if warming protein or veggies)

Total Time: 15–25 min

HOW IT'S GONNA GO DOWN

Grain Prep + Quick Sauté or No-Cook Assembly

BLOCK PARTY (INGREDIENTS)

1. **Grain (½ cup cooked):** Quinoa, brown rice, cauliflower rice, or a ready-made grain mix
2. **Veggies to vibe with (~¾–1 cup total):** Corn, cherry tomatoes, bell pepper, red onion, shredded lettuce, avocado
3. **Sauce/Dressing (~2–3 tbsp):** Salsa, chipotle yogurt, avocado crema, or lime vinaigrette
4. **Optional toppings:** Cilantro, shredded cheese, hot sauce, pico de gallo, sour cream, lime wedge

CALL IN YOUR POWER PLAYERS (~4–6 oz)

- Beans of your choice
- Seasoned ground beef or turkey
- Grilled chicken or shrimp
- Tofu or tempeh

ASSEMBLE YOUR FLAVOR CREW

- **Latin Fiesta:** Cumin, chili powder, onion powder, garlic powder, paprika
  Pairs with: beans, meat, and roasted veggies
- **Southwest Fresh:** Cilantro, lime zest, oregano, chipotle
  Pairs with: corn, quinoa, black beans
- **Zesty & Bright:** Lime juice, avocado oil, red pepper flakes, scallions
  Pairs with: everything

HERE'S THE GAME PLAN – LAYER, DRIZZLE, DIVE IN

1. **Prep grain** (or heat up a pre-cooked/90-second pouch).
2. **Heat a skillet,** add a splash of oil, and brown your protein (if using) if it's not already cooked.
3. **Sprinkle** on your seasoning mix (aka your Flavor Crew) and let it all simmer together for 3–5 minutes. Want more flavor? Toss in the corn for a quick char while you're at it.
4. **In a bowl**, layer your grain, protein, and raw veggies.
5. **Drizzle** with your sauce or dressing of choice — salsa, chipotle yogurt, or whatever you're craving.
6. **Top** with herbs, cheese, crunchy bits — and grab a spoon. Dive in and devour!

PLAY YOUR WILD CARD

- Turn it into tacos or a wrap if you've got tortillas on hand.
- Want crunch? Sprinkle with crushed tortilla chips, toasted nuts, or crispy onions — whatever's in your snack stash.
- Got extras? This one's a leftover MVP — Mix up leftover rice, meat, or veggies for a next-day taco bowl win.

Let's Have a Pep Talk

These stuffed bell peppers are flavor-packed, perfectly portioned, and baked until bubbly. Go meaty, cheesy, or veggie-full — they'll pep up your plate. Once they're in the oven, you've got 30 minutes to chill (PJs optional). And just between us... you might want to make two and win tomorrow's lunch — they reheat like a dream.

Prep Time: 10–15 min

Cook Time: 10 min stovetop, 30–35 min oven

Total Time: 50–60 min

HOW IT'S GONNA GO DOWN

Stovetop Sauté, Simmer & Oven Bake

BLOCK PARTY (INGREDIENTS)

1. **Bell Pepper:** 1 large, top and seeds removed *(chop the top and toss it into the veggie mix)*
2. **Grain or Filler (optional ~½ cup cooked):** Quinoa, rice, lentils, or finely chopped raw cauliflower
3. **Veggies to vibe with (~½–1 cup):** Spinach, mushrooms, tomato, corn, or zucchini
4. **Aromatics (~1 tsp each):** chopped onion, garlic, tomato paste, or ketchup
5. **Cheese (~¼ cup, optional):** Mozzarella, feta, cheddar, or dairy-free shreds
6. **Sauce (~2–3 tbsp):** Tomato sauce, enchilada sauce, pesto, or tahini drizzle

CALL IN YOUR POWER PLAYERS (~4–6 oz)

- ➡ Ground turkey, chicken, or beef
- ➡ Black beans or lentils
- ➡ Plant-based sausage or chopped tofu

ASSEMBLE YOUR FLAVOR CREW

- **Italian Comfort:** Garlic, oregano, basil, thyme
- **Southwest Sizzle:** Cumin, chili powder, paprika
- **Green Goddess:** Parsley, lemon, dill *(great with green veg)*

HERE'S THE GAME PLAN – SIZZLE, STUFF, BAKE, ENJOY

1. **Preheat oven** to 400°F (205°C).
2. **Warm a splash of oil** in a skillet. Add garlic and onion; sauté for 2–3 minutes until softened.
3. **Add your chosen protein**, remaining aromatics, and your flavor crew. If using meat, sauté until fully cooked. For beans or plant-based options, just heat through.
4. **Stir in veggies** and simmer another 3–4 minutes, then mix in your sauce of choice.
5. **Add cooked grain** (if using). Taste and adjust with salt and pepper.
6. **Stuff the bell pepper** tightly with the filling.
7. **Place in a baking dish** and bake uncovered for 20–25 minutes.
8. **Add cheese** (if using) and bake for another 5–10 minutes, until golden and bubbly.
9. **Let cool slightly** before devouring. Want to dress it up? Sprinkle with fresh chopped greens.

PLAY YOUR WILD CARD

- Want a crispier top? Broil for the last 2 minutes.
- No grain? Go low-carb with riced cauliflower or extra veggies.
- Like your pepper crunchy? Just shorten the bake time. For a softer version, give it more oven love.

Shroom for One

A creamy, savory mushroom dish that cooks up in one pot and eats like a hug. Part risotto, part pasta, all comfort — just the right size for a solo treat.

Prep Time: 10 min

Cook Time: 20 min

Total Time: 30 min

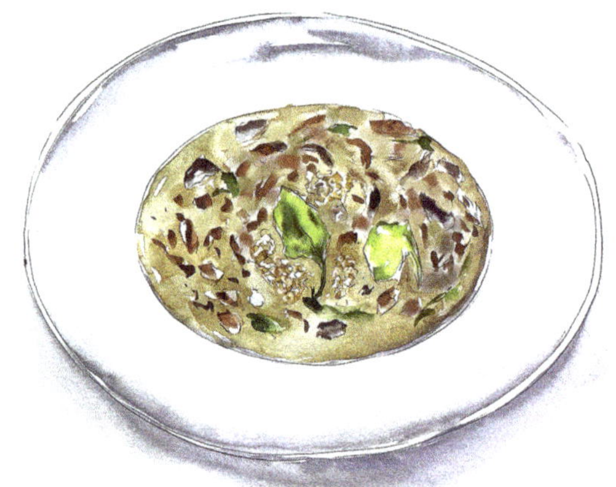

HOW IT'S GONNA GO DOWN

Stovetop Sauté + Simmer

BLOCK PARTY (INGREDIENTS)

Perfect for one filling bowl:

1. **Mushrooms (~1 cup sliced):** Cremini, white button, shiitake — any 'shroom will do.
2. **Aromatics:** ~1 tbsp finely chopped onion or shallot, plus 1 garlic clove (minced)
3. **Grain (~⅓ cup dry):** Orzo (fastest), small pasta, rice, couscous, or quinoa. Note: Some grains (like rice or quinoa) may take a little longer and need a splash more liquid — adjust as needed.
4. **Liquid (~1½, plus more if needed):** Veggie broth, chicken broth, or water
5. **Creamy add-in (optional):** 1–2 tbsp cream cheese, goat cheese, or a splash of milk
6. **Fresh finish (optional):** Lemon zest, Parmesan, parsley, cracked black pepper

CALL IN YOUR POWER PLAYERS (~4 oz)

- Shredded rotisserie chicken
- White beans or chickpeas
- Tofu or tempeh
- Or skip it and let the mushrooms take center stage

ASSEMBLE YOUR FLAVOR CREW

- **French Chic:** Thyme, parsley, cracked pepper, splash of white wine. Top with: goat cheese + lemon zest
- **Earthy Umami:** Garlic, soy sauce, miso paste, sesame oil
  Great with: tofu + scallions
- **Cozy Comfort:** Paprika, oregano, Parmesan, butter
  Great with: chicken or beans

HERE'S THE GAME PLAN – SAUTÉ, SIMMER, STIR

1. **In a small pot, sauté aromatics** in oil or butter for 2–3 minutes.
2. **Add mushrooms** and cook until golden and fragrant (5–6 min).
3. **Stir in your grain**, any cooked or ready-to-eat protein (if using), flavor crew, and broth (start with 1½ cups).
4. **Simmer uncovered**, stirring occasionally, until the grain is tender and liquid is mostly absorbed (about 15–18 min).
5. **Stir in your creamy element** (if using), finish with fresh herbs or cheese, and dive in — straight from the pot if you're feelin' it.

PLAY YOUR WILD CARD

- Want greens? Toss in a handful of spinach or arugula in the last 2 minutes.
- Prefer it soupier? Add a splash more broth at the end.
- Cozy vibes? A hunk of crusty bread or a glass of wine turns this into a next-level solo feast.

Eggs in a Hot Tub

Eggs fried in a spiced tomato and veggie sauce — rich, vibrant, and ready to scoop straight from the pan. It's fast, fancy-feeling, and exactly what happens when your eggs decide to kick back and simmer in style. So, go ahead — crack an egg, claim your skillet, and let the steamy magic happen.

Prep Time: 10 min

Cook Time: 15–20 min

Total Time: 25–30 min

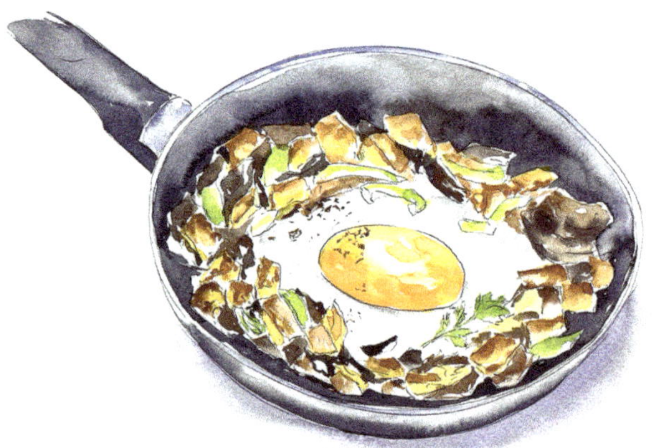

HOW IT'S GONNA GO DOWN

Stovetop Simmer

BLOCK PARTY (INGREDIENTS)

Perfect for one satisfying meal.

1. **Eggs:** 1–2 large
2. **Veggies to vibe with (~½–¾ cup):** Bell pepper, spinach, zucchini, green beans, potatoes
3. **Aromatics:** ~1 tsp garlic, 2–3 tsp chopped onion, a pinch of chili flakes, cumin, paprika, and ~1 tsp tomato or harissa paste
4. **Saucy base (~1½ cups):** Crushed tomatoes or canned diced tomatoes (lightly drained), plus a splash of water
5. **Optional toppings:** Feta, parsley or cilantro, toasted bread, yogurt dollop

CALL IN YOUR POWER PLAYERS (optional)

- Eggs are the main event here — but if you want to bulk it up:
- Chickpeas or beans for extra body
- Crumbled sausage or leftover chicken for a heartier dish
- Or go full veg — it's plenty satisfying on its own

ASSEMBLE YOUR FLAVOR CREW

- **Spicy & Smoky:** Cumin, paprika, chili flakes, garlic
  Top with: feta + parsley
- **Herby & Fresh:** Thyme, oregano, basil
  Top with: goat cheese or fresh greens.
- **Garlic Lover's Delight:** Extra garlic, black pepper, lemon zest
  Drizzle with: olive oil and yogurt

HERE'S THE GAME PLAN – SIMMER, CRACK, SCOOP

1. **Heat oil in a skillet.** Sauté garlic and onion for 1–2 minutes.
2. **Add veggies** and cook until softened (6-8 minutes, potatoes might take a bit longer).
3. **Stir in sausage** (if using), sauce base, and remaining aromatics + flavor crew. Simmer until slightly thickened (5–8 minutes).
4. **Make one or two little wells** in the sauce, add a little oil or butter into each, and crack an egg into each well. Season with salt and pepper.
5. **Cover and cook gently** until the whites are set and the yolks are done to your liking (5–7 minutes).
6. **Remove from heat** and top with whatever you love — herbs, cheese, toast, or creamy extras.

PLAY YOUR WILD CARD

- Want to skip the eggs? Add white beans for a plant-based twist.
- Feeling brunchy? Serve over fresh pita or crusty bread with a dollop of lemony yogurt or avocado slices.
- Craving more heat? Drizzle your favorite hot sauce over the top.

Bangkok in a Pan

This Thai-inspired skillet brings the sweet, salty, spicy, and tangy straight to your stovetop — no passport required. With tofu, chicken, shrimp, or just veg, it's your one-pan ticket to bold flavor and zero effort. Quick, flexible, and totally wokin' it.

Prep Time: 10–15 min

Cook Time: 15 min

Total Time: 25–30 min

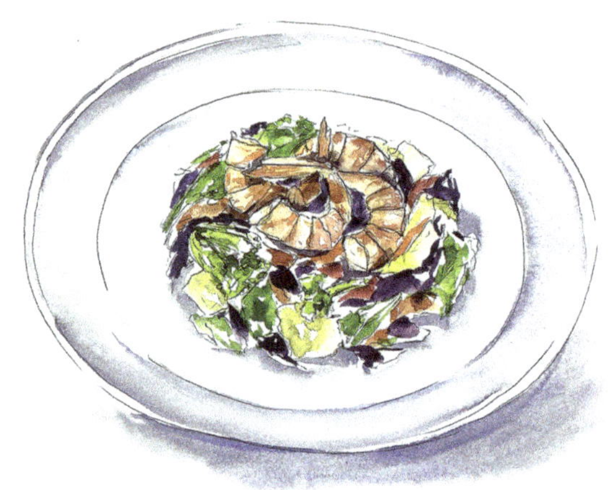

HOW IT'S GONNA GO DOWN

Stovetop Stir-Fry

BLOCK PARTY (INGREDIENTS)

This builds one generous serving.

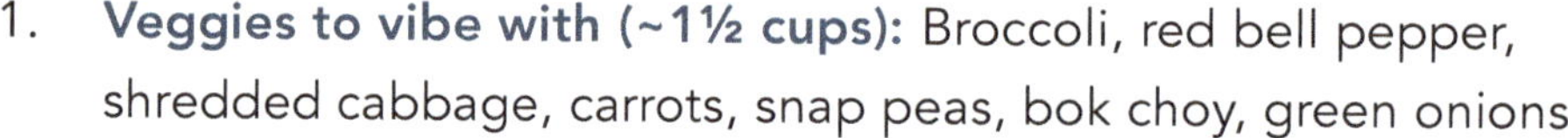

1. **Veggies to vibe with (~1½ cups):** Broccoli, red bell pepper, shredded cabbage, carrots, snap peas, bok choy, green onions
2. **Aromatics:** ~1 tsp each minced garlic and ginger, a pinch of red chili flakes or fresh chili
3. **Sauce (~2–3 tbsp):** Peanut sauce*, or Thai curry paste + coconut milk, or soy sauce + lime + honey + garlic **See easy homemade peanut sauce in the back!*
4. **Oil (~1 tsp):** Coconut oil, sesame oil, or avocado oil

CALL IN YOUR POWER PLAYERS (~4–6 oz)

- Chicken or pork (sliced thin)
- Shrimp
- Tofu (firm, pan-seared)
- Tempeh or chickpeas

ASSEMBLE YOUR FLAVOR CREW

- **Sweet & Nutty:** Peanut sauce, chili flakes, lime juice
  Top with: crushed peanuts + cilantro
- **Coconut Curry:** Red curry paste, garlic, ginger, coconut milk
  Finish with: Thai basil or lime zest
- **Zesty Garlic Soy:** Soy sauce, lime juice, honey, garlic
  Top with: green onion + sesame seeds

HERE'S THE GAME PLAN – SIZZLE & SAUCE

1. **Heat oil in a skillet** over medium-high.
2. **Add your protein** and sear until golden and cooked through (~5–6 min). Remove and set aside.
3. **In the same skillet, stir-fry veggies** and aromatics for 4–5 minutes, until crisp-tender.
4. **Return protein to the pan**. Add sauce and your flavor crew. Toss to coat everything evenly.
5. **Simmer for 2–3 minutes** to bring it all together.
6. **Taste, adjust** — a splash more spice, soy, or citrus if needed. Serve hot, right from the skillet.

PLAY YOUR WILD CARD

- Want it saucier? Add a splash of broth or extra coconut milk.
- Craving carbs? Toss in some leftover rice or noodles.
- Bonus points for topping with a lime wedge, scallions, or sesame crunch.

Mac My Day

A skillet mac-and-cheese crafted for solo indulgence—creamy, cheesy, and anything but basic. This leveled-up version lets you toss in your favorite veggies, protein, and a crunchy topping (if that's your thing). Endlessly customizable and made in one pot, this dish will totally mac your day—comfort food, redefined.

Prep Time: 10 min

Cook Time: 15–20 min

Total Time: 25–30 min

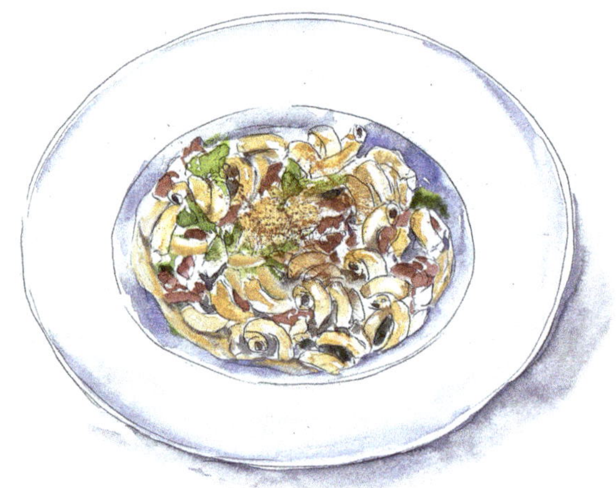

HOW IT'S GONNA GO DOWN

Stovetop Boil + Skillet Stir

BLOCK PARTY (INGREDIENTS)

Makes one hearty serving:

1. **Pasta (~¾ cup dry / ~1½ cups cooked):** Elbows, shells, penne, or GF pasta
2. **Liquid (~½ cup):** Milk, plant milk, or a splash of cream (whatever you've got)
3. **Cheese (~⅓–½ cup shredded):** Cheddar, mozzarella, Parmesan, or a mix
4. **Veggies to vibe with (optional) (~½ cup):** Spinach, peas, broccoli or roasted veggies
5. **Crunchy topping (optional):** 1 tbsp breadcrumbs toasted in oil or butter

CALL IN YOUR POWER PLAYERS (~4 oz)

- Diced ham or cooked chicken
- Crumbled sausage or bacon bits
- White beans or green peas
- Keep it classic with just the cheese

"Mac + your favorite extras = pure magic, no matter the day."

ASSEMBLE YOUR FLAVOR CREW

- **Classic Comfort**: Salt, pepper, garlic powder, paprika
  Top with: breadcrumbs + a sprinkle of love
- **Zesty Kick**: Cayenne, chili flakes, smoked paprika, chipotle cheese. Finish with: hot sauce or jalapeños
- **Herby Deluxe**:
  Thyme, chives, parsley, lemon zest
  Great with: spinach, peas, or light protein

HERE'S THE GAME PLAN – BOIL, STIR, CREAMIFY

1. **Cook pasta** in salted water until just tender. Drain and set aside.
2. **In the same pot, melt butter or oil**, add veggies (if using) and cook until done to your liking. No veggies? No problem — just move to the next step.
3. **Add liquid** and bring to a gentle simmer. Stir in shredded cheese and your flavor crew until melted and smooth.
4. **Add pasta** and any extras (ready-to-eat protein). Stir to coat it all in creamy goodness.
5. **Let it simmer on low for 2–3 min** until everything is hot and velvety.
6. **Top with breadcrumbs or extra cheese** if you're feeling fancy. Serve hot.

PLAY YOUR WILD CARD

- No milk? Use pasta water with a bit of butter and cheese — works like a charm.
- Want a crusty top? Slide it under the broiler for 2-3 minutes (just watch it!).
- Leftovers? Not likely… but if so, reheat gently with a splash of liquid.

Bake It Till You Make It

This one-pan wonder roasts your whole dinner in one go — protein, veg, the whole shebang. You'll get golden edges, juicy bites, and bold flavor with barely any cleanup (parchment paper to the rescue!). No stress, no fuss. Just pop it in the oven and let it do the heavy lifting.

Prep Time: 10 min

Cook Time: 15–20 min

Total Time: 25–30 min

HOW IT'S GONNA GO DOWN

Sheet Pan Roast

BLOCK PARTY (INGREDIENTS)

Makes one complete meal — protein + veggies, all on one sheet pan.

1. **Veggies to vibe with (~1½ cups):** Broccoli, asparagus, green beans, cherry tomatoes, bell pepper, baby potatoes
2. **Aromatics:** A pinch or two each: salt, pepper, garlic powder, lemon zest
3. **Acid:** Juice of ½ lemon or a splash of vinegar

CALL IN YOUR POWER PLAYERS (~4-6 oz)

- ➡ White fish, like cod or tilapia (fresh or thawed, skin-on or off)
- ➡ Salmon fillet (fresh or thawed, skin-on or off)
- ➡ Tofu (pressed + sliced thick)
- ➡ Tempeh or chickpeas

*"Not into fish?
Your oven doesn't care —
this method works
for lots of proteins."*

ASSEMBLE YOUR FLAVOR CREW

- **Lemon-Herb:** Thyme, garlic, parsley, lemon zest
  Top with: lemon slice + drizzle of olive oil
- **Spicy Citrus:** Chili flakes, smoked paprika, lime juice
  Top with: hot honey or chili crisp
- **Garlic Butter Vibes:** Garlic powder, rosemary, butter
  Top with: a squeeze of lemon or fresh herbs

HERE'S THE GAME PLAN – ROAST & RELAX

1. **Preheat oven** to 400°F (200°C).
2. **Toss chopped veggies** with a splash of oil and your flavor crew. Spread them on one half of a sheet pan (don't crowd them — they'll crisp up better that way).
3. **Place your protein** on the other half. Drizzle with oil and sprinkle with aromatics. Top with lemon slices or extra seasoning.
4. **Roast for 15–20 minutes**, until veggies are tender and protein is fully cooked (fish should flake easily with a fork).
5. **Finish with a squeeze of lemon** and serve straight from the pan — zero drama, all flavor.

PLAY YOUR WILD CARD

- Want crispy edges? Broil for the last 2–3 minutes.
- Fancy it up? Add a dollop of yogurt, pesto, or garlic aioli.
- Keep it simple. This meal is complete as-is — no sides needed (though a glass of wine wouldn't hurt).

Veggies Gone Wild

This isn't your average grain bowl — this is what happens when roasted veggies turn up the heat and steal the spotlight. Sweet, savory, herby, and totally over the top (in the best way). It's a full-on flavor bomb, and your mouth better be ready.

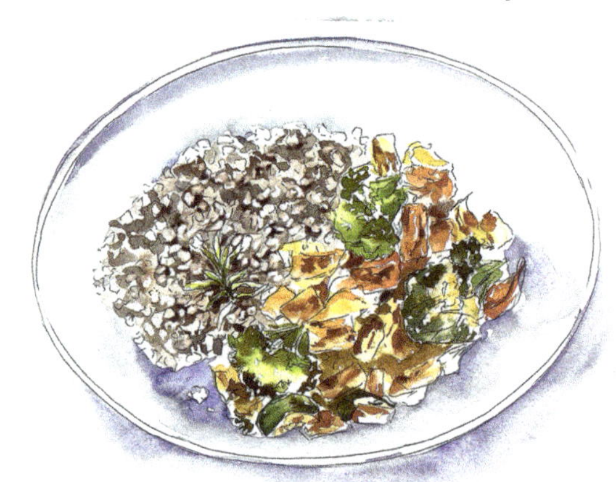

Prep Time: 10–15 min

Cook Time: 20–25 min

Total Time: 30–35 min

HOW IT'S GONNA GO DOWN

Sheet Pan Roast + Bowl Assembly

BLOCK PARTY (INGREDIENTS)

Makes 1 warm, satisfying bowl of goodness.

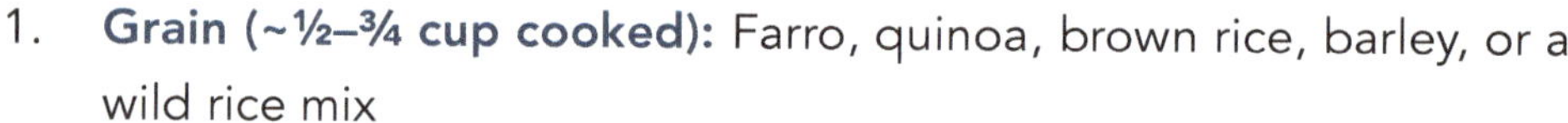

1. **Grain (~½–¾ cup cooked):** Farro, quinoa, brown rice, barley, or a wild rice mix
2. **Veggies to vibe with (~1–1½ cups chopped):** Potatoes (any kind), zucchini, cauliflower, red onion, carrots, beets, turnips, pumpkin, squash, Brussels sprouts, broccoli — seriously, everything goes here
3. **Aromatics:** Pinch each of salt, pepper, and your chosen Flavor Crew seasonings
4. **Optional Toppings:** Feta, goat cheese, tahini, toasted nuts, or fresh herbs

CALL IN YOUR POWER PLAYERS (~4–6 oz)

- Roasted or sautéed chickpeas
- Grilled or pre-cooked chicken or tofu
- White beans or tempeh (no extra cooking needed)
- Or go all-veg and let the grain + toppings take the lead...

ASSEMBLE YOUR FLAVOR CREW

- **Cozy & Earthy:** Rosemary, thyme, garlic powder, black pepper
  Great with: sweet potato, beets, farro
- **Lemon-Herb Fresh:** Parsley, dill, lemon zest, squeeze of juice
  Great with: quinoa, tofu, and feta
- **Bold & Smoky:** Smoked paprika, cumin, chili flakes, olive oil
  Great with: chickpeas, cauliflower, tahini drizzle

HERE'S THE GAME PLAN – ROAST, BUILD, ENJOY

1. **Preheat oven** to 400°F (200°C).
2. **Toss chopped veggies** (and any protein that needs cooking — like tofu or raw tempeh) with oil and your flavor crew seasonings. Spread evenly on a parchment-lined baking sheet for easy cleanup.
3. **Roast for 20–25 minutes**, flipping halfway through for even golden deliciousness.
4. **While that's happening, warm your grain** or grab it pre-cooked from the fridge.
5. **Layer** grain in your bowl, pile on those roasted beauties, and finish with toppings like feta, herbs, or a dreamy drizzle.
6. **Take a victory bite** — you just built a bowl that slaps.

PLAY YOUR WILD CARD

- Want it creamy? Add a scoop of hummus or tahini-yogurt drizzle.
- Short on time? Use pre-chopped veggies or yesterday's roasted leftovers.
- Travels well! Perfect warm or at room temp — meal prep approved.

Egg-cuse Me, Dinner?

This crispy, one-pan hash is your permission slip to eat breakfast for dinner — or whenever the heck you want. Golden potatoes, savory mix-ins, and an egg on top (because obviously). Toss in whatever you've got — this dish doesn't judge, it just shows up and sizzles.

Prep Time: 10 min

Cook Time: 15–20 min

Total Time: 25–30 min

HOW IT'S GONNA GO DOWN

Stovetop Skillet Sizzle

BLOCK PARTY (INGREDIENTS)

Makes one skillet-full of golden goodness.

1. **Potatoes (~1 cup, diced small):** Yukon gold, red, or sweet potatoes — peeled or not
2. **Veggies to vibe with (~½–¾ cup):** Bell pepper, onion, spinach, mushrooms, zucchini
3. **Aromatics:** 1–2 tsp minced garlic, chopped scallions, or shallots.
4. **Egg (optional):** 1–2 eggs, fried or scrambled right into the pan

CALL IN YOUR POWER PLAYERS (~4-6 oz cooked)

- Diced sausage or bacon
- Tofu, tempeh, or black beans
- Leftover steak, chicken, or veggie burger
- Or go all veg — it still hits

"This is your clean-out-the-fridge hero disguised as a diner favorite."

ASSEMBLE YOUR FLAVOR CREW

- **Classic Diner:** Paprika, garlic powder, onion powder, parsley
  Top with: Ketchup or hot sauce
- **Spicy Southwest:** Cumin, chili powder, jalapeños
  Top with: Avocado, salsa, lime
- **Fresh & Green:** Thyme, rosemary, chives, lemon zest
  Top with: Poached egg + greens

HERE'S THE GAME PLAN – CRISP, FLIP, CRACK

1. **Heat oil in a skillet**. Add diced potatoes and cook over medium heat, flipping occasionally until golden and fork-tender (about 10–12 minutes).
2. **Toss in veggies**, aromatics, and flavor crew. Stir and cook until softened and slightly charred (about 5–7 minutes).
3. **Add cooked protein** if using. Stir to combine.
4. **Crack eggs directly into the pan** and let them cook to your liking, or fry separately and serve on top.
5. **Season well** and serve hot — crispy edges are the goal.

PLAY YOUR WILD CARD

- Want it cheesy? Stir in a little shredded cheddar or goat cheese at the end.
- Sweet potatoes make it feel special — and they crisp like a dream.
- Top with hot sauce, salsa, or a spoonful of sour cream if you're feelin' it.

Frittata Me Not

Savory, sassy, and just bougie enough — these mini solo frittatas bring the flavor without the fuss. Whether you're going meaty, cheesy, veggie, or all three, they're your ticket to baked egg brilliance.

Prep Time: 10 min

Cook Time: 15–20 min

Total Time: 25–30 min

HOW IT'S GONNA GO DOWN

Oven Bake (Muffin Tin or Ramekins)

BLOCK PARTY (INGREDIENTS)

Makes 2–3 mini frittatas (depending on size of your muffin tin or ramekin).

1. **Eggs:** 2–3 large
2. **Veggies to vibe with (~½–1 cup):** Spinach, bell pepper, onion, mushrooms, tomato
3. **Creamy add-in (optional):** 1–2 tbsp milk, cream, or plain yogurt
4. **Cheese (~2–3 tbsp):** Feta, cheddar, goat cheese, or mozzarella

CALL IN YOUR POWER PLAYERS (~2–4 oz)

- ➟ Diced ham or cooked bacon
- ➟ Crumbled sausage (meat or plant-based)
- ➟ Tofu crumbles

ASSEMBLE YOUR FLAVOR CREW

- **Mediterranean Morning:** Oregano, basil, sun-dried tomato, feta
  Top with: fresh parsley
- **Wake Me Up:** Smoked paprika, chili flakes, sharp cheddar
  Top with: hot sauce or salsa
- **Garden Fresh:** Thyme, chives, spinach, goat cheese
  Top with: lemon zest or arugula

HERE'S THE GAME PLAN – WHISK, FILL, BAKE

1. **Preheat oven** to 375°F (190°C). Grease 2 muffin cups or 1-2 small ramekins, depending on your batch size.
2. **Whisk eggs** with salt, pepper, and creamy add-in (if using).
3. **Stir in chopped veggies**, protein, cheese, and your Flavor Crew seasonings.
4. **Pour into prepared cups**, filling about ¾ full.
5. **Bake for 15–20 minutes**, until puffed and set.
6. **Let cool slightly** — they might deflate a bit, but the flavor stays bold and beautiful.

PLAY YOUR WILD CARD

- Great warm or cold — leftovers make a killer breakfast, lunch, or snack.
- Feeling creative? Line muffin cups with a slice of ham or tortilla for a built-in "crust."
- Hot to trot? Drizzle with hot sauce or serve with salsa and a dollop of sour cream.
- Pair with a side salad, toast, or fruit if you're feeling extra.

Umami in a Hurry

This savory rice bowl pulls no punches — it owns the whole flavor map. Grains, greens, and whatever protein's making eyes at you from the fridge. Hot, cold, or somewhere in between — it's got solo dinner written all over it. A quick stir, a bold glaze, and boom: dinner with attitude, all in one bowl.

Prep Time: 10–15 min

Cook Time: 5–10 min (if sautéing anything)

Total Time: 15–25 min

HOW IT'S GONNA GO DOWN

Grain Prep + Quick Sauté or No-Cook Assembly

BLOCK PARTY (INGREDIENTS)

This makes one full bowl of umami goodness.

1. **Grain (~½ cup cooked):** Any type of rice, orzo, couscous, quinoa, or a ready-to-eat pouch
2. **Veggies to vibe with (~¾–1 cup):** Carrots, cherry tomatoes, kale, roasted sweet potato, corn — whatever's calling your name
3. **Sauce (~2–3 tbsp):** Soy sauce or tamari, mirin or honey, garlic, + a drizzle of sesame oil
   (Tamari brings richer, deeper umami and is less salty)
4. **Optional toppings:** Seaweed flakes, chili flakes, toasted sesame, avocado slice

CALL IN YOUR POWER PLAYERS (~4–6 oz)

- Chicken, pork, or beef
- Seared tofu
- Pan-fried salmon or shrimp
- Tempeh, edamame, or even a hard-boiled egg

"This bowl loves leftovers — or a quick sizzle in the skillet."

ASSEMBLE YOUR FLAVOR CREW

- **Teriyaki Vibes:** Soy sauce + honey + garlic + sesame oil
  Top with: Sesame seeds + scallions
- **Spicy-Sweet Kick:** Ginger, garlic, sriracha or gochujang, maple syrup, mirin
  Top with: Chili flakes + avocado
- **Light & Fresh:** Ponzu, lime, cucumber, seaweed
  Top with: Pickled ginger + a splash of rice vinegar

HERE'S THE GAME PLAN – STIR, SIZZLE, STACK

1. **Cook or warm your grain**.
2. **In a skillet, cook protein** (if raw) in a splash of oil until nearly done.
3. **Add any veggies** that need cooking and sauté to your preferred doneness.
4. **Make your sauce**: Mix sauce ingredients in a small bowl.
5. **Build your bowl**: Grain first, then veggies, protein, sauce, and finally toppings.
6. **Sit back and enjoy** your umami masterpiece.

PLAY YOUR WILD CARD

- Add crunch: Nuts, seeds, or crumbled cheese.
- Swap grain for noodles if you're feeling noodly.
- Keep it raw or sautéed — either way, you've got a full plate in a bowl.

Holy Frijole

This Latin-inspired bowl is stacked with spiced beans, roasted sweet potato, creamy avocado, and a zesty lime drizzle — all over warm rice or quinoa. It's colorful, comforting, and way too flavorful to keep quiet about. One bite and you'll enter Holy Frijole land.

Prep Time: 10–15 min

Cook Time: 15–20 min

Total Time: 25–30 min

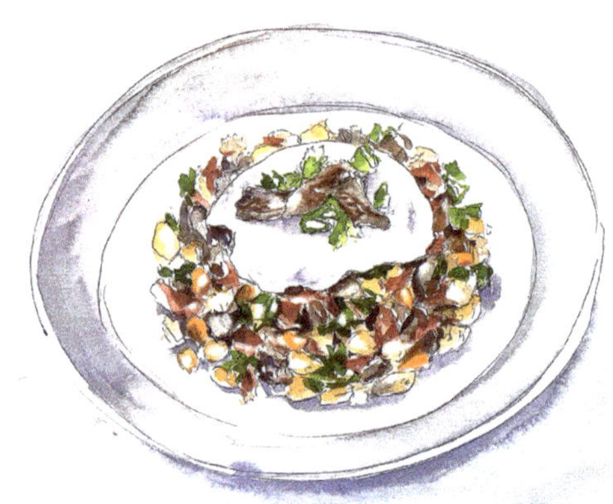

HOW IT'S GONNA GO DOWN

Skillet Simmer

BLOCK PARTY (INGREDIENTS)

This makes one full-flavored bowl of goodness.

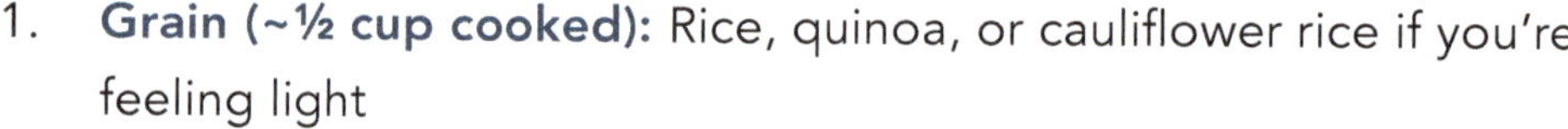

1. **Grain (~½ cup cooked):** Rice, quinoa, or cauliflower rice if you're feeling light
2. **Beans (~½ can, drained):** Black, pinto, or red — your call
3. **Veggies (~1–1½ cups cubed):** Sweet potato, corn, bell pepper, red onion
4. **Aromatics:** ~1–1½ tsp each: minced garlic & finely chopped onion plus a sprinkle of cumin
5. **Sauce or drizzle (~2 tbsp):** Lime crema (below — trust me, it's delish), chipotle mayo, or avocado crema

CALL IN YOUR POWER PLAYERS (~4–6 oz)

- ➡ Beans as main (keep it veggie!)
- ➡ Shredded rotisserie chicken
- ➡ Chorizo or ground turkey
- ➡ Plant-based ground or grilled tofu

ASSEMBLE YOUR FLAVOR CREW

- **Chipotle Bold:** Smoked paprika, cumin, garlic, chili powder
  Drizzle with: chipotle mayo or lime crema
- **Sweet & Spiced:** Cinnamon, cumin, smoked salt
  Great with: roasted sweet potato + beans
- **Fresh & Bright:** Cilantro, lime zest, oregano, jalapeño
  Top with: scallions, lime juice, avocado

HERE'S THE GAME PLAN – SAUTÉ, STIR, STACK

1. **Cook your protein** in a bit of oil with seasoning. Set aside once done. *(Skip if using precooked protein.)*
2. **In the same skillet,** sauté veggies with oil, aromatics, and your flavor crew for 10–15 minutes, until golden and tender.
3. **Add beans** and sauté another 4–5 minutes, until everything's cozy and coated in flavor.
4. **Warm your grain** if you want, or keep it cold — it's a bowl, not a rule.
5. **Build your bowl:** grain → veggie + beans → protein → drizzle → toppings.
6. **Top** with avocado slices, cilantro, scallions, or lime wedges.

PLAY YOUR WILD CARD

- Want crunch? Top with tortilla strips, plantain chips, or even a pork rind (like I did).
- Feeling saucy? Hit it with a generous drizzle of lime crema (below).
- Add heat with jalapeño slices, hot sauce, or salsa.

LIME CREMA (QUICK SAUCE)

- 2 tbsp sour cream or Greek yogurt
- Zest + juice of ½ lime
- Pinch of garlic powder + salt. Mix well and drizzle or dollop as desired.

Wrap Me Baby One More Time

This warm, flavor-packed tortilla is stuffed with spiced protein, crunchy veggies, and a creamy drizzle that hits all the right notes. Fold it, roll it, devour it — this wrap's got solo dinner on repeat.

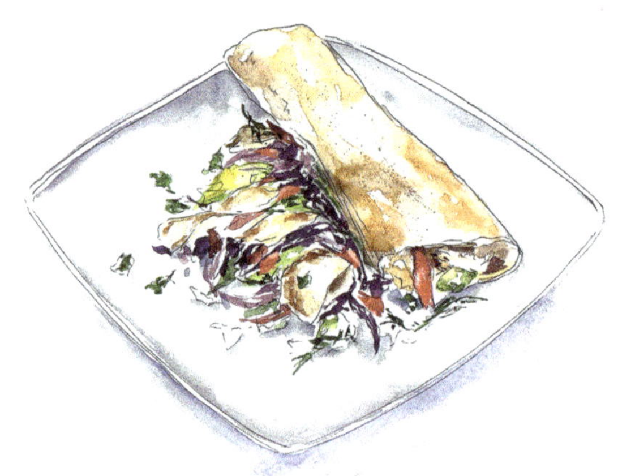

Prep Time: 10 min

Cook Time: 10–15 min

Total Time: 20–25 min

HOW IT'S GONNA GO DOWN

Stovetop Sear + Quick Assembly

BLOCK PARTY (INGREDIENTS)

Build one perfect wrap (or two lighter ones).

1. **Tortilla or wrap base**: 8–10-inch flour, whole wheat, GF tortilla, or collard green leaf
2. **Veggies (~¾ cup total)**: Lettuce, cabbage slaw, tomatoes, red onion, bell peppers, corn, avocado
3. **Sauce (~2–3 tbsp)**: Chipotle mayo, garlic yogurt, lime crema, tahini

CALL IN YOUR POWER PLAYERS (~4–6 oz)

- ➟ Seasoned chicken or shrimp
- ➟ Sautéed black beans + onions
- ➟ Crispy tofu strips or grilled tempeh
- ➟ Leftover taco meat, steak, or rotisserie chicken

"If it fits in a tortilla, it belongs in this wrap."

ASSEMBLE YOUR FLAVOR CREW

- **Taco Tuesday**: Cumin, chili powder, paprika, garlic
  Top with: salsa, avocado, lime
- **Street Style**: Smoked paprika, chipotle, onion powder
  Top with: hot sauce + crema
- **Garden Crunch**: Lemon zest, dill, cucumber, hummus
  Top with: greens + pickled red onions

HERE'S THE GAME PLAN – SIZZLE, STACK, ROLL

1. **Warm tortilla** in a skillet or microwave until soft and pliable. If using a collard green leaf, remove the tick stem and massage it to make it easier to roll.
2. **If using raw protein**, sear it first with oil and your flavor crew, then let the veggies crash the party for the last few minutes.
3. **Spread your sauce** across the tortilla (or collard leaf).
4. **Add veggies**, cooked protein, and any extras.
5. **Fold in the sides**, then roll it up from the bottom. Slice in half if you're feeling fancy.

PLAY YOUR WILD CARD

- No wrap? Turn it into a bowl with the same ingredients over rice or quinoa.
- Want extra crunch? Add crushed chips or slaw inside.
- These wrap beautifully for lunch tomorrow — just leave off wet ingredients until serving.

LIME CREMA (QUICK SAUCE)

- 2 tbsp sour cream or Greek yogurt
- Zest + juice of ½ lime
- Pinch of garlic powder + salt. Mix well and drizzle or dollop as desired.

Crust Me, It's Good

Toasty bread, melty cheese, and your choice of savory toppings — all broiled to bubbly perfection. It's quick, comforting, and just elevated enough to feel like you made an effort… even if you didn't. Warning: you may want to make another one immediately.

Prep Time: 10 min

Cook Time: 5–7 min (under the broiler)

Total Time: 15–17 min

HOW IT'S GONNA GO DOWN

Broiler + Light Mixing

BLOCK PARTY (INGREDIENTS)

Makes 1 large open-faced sandwich (or 2 minis).

1. **Bread base:** 1 thick slice sourdough, rye, multigrain, or GF bread
2. **Veggies to vibe with (~½ cup):** Finely chopped tomato, pickles, olives, scallions, onions, or celery
3. **Aromatics:** ~½ tsp Dijon or grainy mustard, salt, and pepper
4. **Fat:** ~1 tbsp mayo, plain yogurt, or mashed avocado
5. **Cheese (~2 tbsp shredded or sliced):** Cheddar, Swiss, mozzarella, or dairy-free
6. **Drizzle or crunch (optional):** Chili crisp, hot honey, or a sprinkle of everything bagel seasoning

CALL IN YOUR POWER PLAYERS (~4–6 oz)

- Canned tuna or chicken (drained)
- Shredded rotisserie chicken
- Smashed white beans or chickpeas
- Smoked salmon + herbed goat cheese for a fancy flair

ASSEMBLE YOUR FLAVOR CREW

- **Deli Classic:** Dijon, cracked pepper, red onion
  Top with: cheddar + tomato
- **Zesty Heat:** Chili flakes, jalapeño, spicy mayo
  Top with: chipotle jack cheese + scallions
- **Mediterranean:** Lemon zest, oregano, kalamata olives
  Top with: mozzarella or feta + sliced tomato

HERE'S THE GAME PLAN – MIX, MELT, MUNCH

1. **Preheat broiler** to low. Lightly toast bread (1–2 min — watch it!).
2. **In a bowl, mix** protein, veggies, fat, aromatics, and flavor crew (if using).
3. **Taste and adjust** mixture to your liking.
4. **Spread mixture** onto toasted bread. Top with cheese and extras.
5. **Broil 2–4 minutes**, until cheese is bubbly and golden.
6. **Let cool 1–2 minutes**. Slice it up — or just grab and go.

PLAY YOUR WILD CARD

- Want extra crunch? Add crushed chips or breadcrumbs before broiling.
- Use English muffins or mini naan for cute, personal-size melts.
- Serve with a simple salad or pickled veggies for a full diner-style experience.

Flavor Jacuzzi

Get ready to take your taste buds for a soak in this spicy, steamy, flavor-packed broth. It's cozy, it's got kick, and it's the most delicious Jacuzzi you've ever dipped a spoon into.

Prep Time: 10 min

Cook Time: 10–15 min

Total Time: 20–25 min

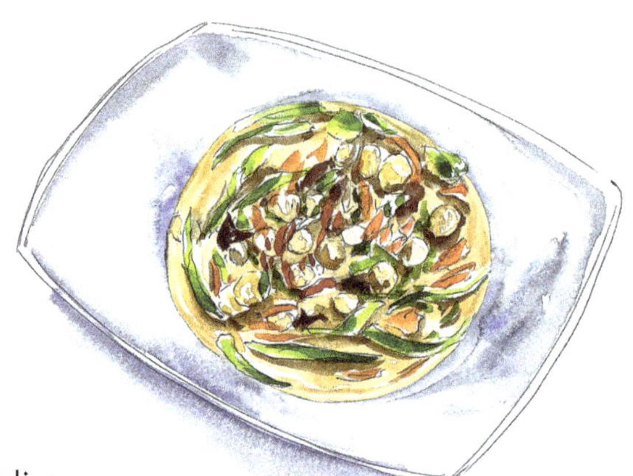

HOW IT'S GONNA GO DOWN

Stovetop Sauté + Simmer

BLOCK PARTY (INGREDIENTS)

This makes one full bowl of broth-based bliss.

1. **Noodles (~2 oz dry):** Ramen, soba, rice noodles, or spaghetti
2. **Broth (~1½ cups):** Veggie, chicken, or miso — add a splash of coconut milk for extra creaminess
3. **Veggies to vibe with (~1 cup):** Bok choy, spinach, mushrooms, shredded carrots, snow peas, scallions
4. **Aromatics:** ~½ tsp each minced or finely sliced garlic, ginger, green onion
5. **Toppings (optional but fabulous):** Soft-boiled egg, chili oil, sesame seeds, lime wedge, fresh herbs *(like basil, cilantro, or scallions — whatever you've got)*

CALL IN YOUR POWER PLAYERS (~4–6 oz)

- Sliced chicken breast or thighs
- Shrimp or tofu cubes
- Boiled egg or edamame
- Leftover roast pork or rotisserie chicken
- Chickpeas (½ can, drained)

"This bowl is all about balance — hot broth, tender veg, a little chew, and lots of cozy."

ASSEMBLE YOUR FLAVOR CREW

- **Miso Magic:** Miso paste + soy sauce + sesame oil
  Great with: tofu, mushrooms, greens
- **Spicy Ginger-Garlic:** Chili flakes + fresh ginger + lime juice
  Great with: chicken, bok choy, carrots
- **Clean & Green:** Lemon zest, cilantro, garlic, scallions
  Top with: lime, fresh herbs, drizzle of olive oil

HERE'S THE GAME PLAN – SIMMER, SLURP, SMILE

1. **Cook noodles** according to package. Drain and set aside in a strainer.
2. **In the same pot** (because why dirty another one?), heat a little oil and sauté your aromatics for 2 minutes. Yep, your pot's pulling double duty — just the way we like it.
3. **Add your protein** and cook through if raw, then set aside. If it's already cooked, toss it in later with the noodles so it doesn't get rubbery.
4. **Stir in your veggies**, broth, and flavor crew. Simmer until everything's steamy and dreamy (5–7 min).
5. **Toss the noodles** back in for a quick warm-up (1–2 min). Taste and adjust seasoning.
6. **Pour into your favorite bowl**, pile on the toppings, and slurp away.

PLAY YOUR WILD CARD

- Swap noodles for spiralized zucchini or cabbage strips for a low-carb vibe. No cooking needed — just toss 'em in with your hot veggies.
- Use frozen veggie mixes or leftover roasted veggies to save time.
- No noodles? Leftover rice works like a charm — soak it up and slurp it down.

Tossed and Sauced

A one-pan pasta (or rice) dish that comes together fast with just a handful of ingredients and a whole lotta flavor. Garlic, herbs, olive oil, and your favorite mix-ins — tossed, sauced, and so satisfying you'll want it again tomorrow.

Prep Time: 5–10 min

Cook Time: 15–20 min

Total Time: 20–30 min

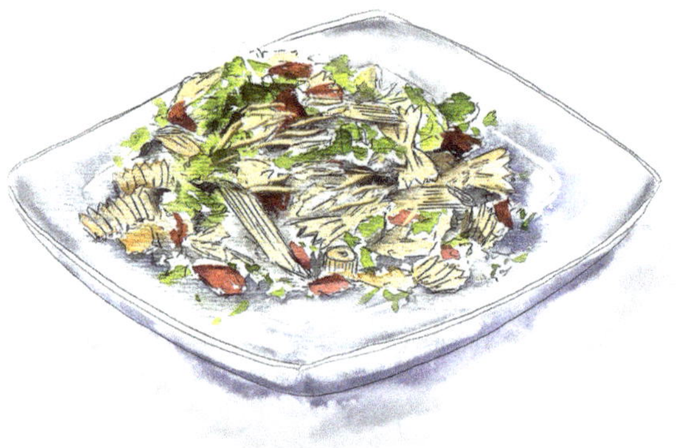

HOW IT'S GONNA GO DOWN

Stovetop Boil + Toss in Skillet

BLOCK PARTY (INGREDIENTS)

One serving of pasta perfection.

1. **Pasta (~¾ cup dry / ~1½ cups cooked):** Spaghetti, penne, fusilli, macaroni, or gluten-free pasta
2. **Sauce base (~2–3 tbsp):** Olive oil, butter, or both — your skillet, your rules
3. **Aromatics:** 1 garlic clove minced, red pepper flakes (optional), lemon zest (optional)
4. **Veggies to vibe with (~½–1 cup):** Cherry tomatoes, spinach, olives, roasted red peppers, artichokes, zucchini
5. **Cheese (optional):** Parmesan, goat cheese, feta, or dairy-free alternative

"The secret sauce here is… actually the sauce. Toss, taste, tweak. You can't mess this up."

CALL IN YOUR POWER PLAYERS (~4 oz)

- Grilled chicken
- Shrimp or tuna
- White beans or chickpeas
- Or go full veg — the oil + cheese combo totally delivers

ASSEMBLE YOUR FLAVOR CREW

- **Classic Italiano:** Garlic, chili flakes, parsley, olive oil
  Top with: Parmesan + lemon juice
- **Herby & Bright:** Fresh herbs, garlic, lemon
  Top with: goat cheese + pine nuts
- **Bold & Saucy:** Sun-dried tomato pesto, olives, paprika, chili flakes
  Top with: feta or mozzarella pearls

HERE'S THE GAME PLAN – BOIL, SIZZLE, TOSS

1. **Cook pasta** in salted water. Save ¼ cup pasta water before draining.
2. **While pasta cooks**, warm oil or butter in a skillet with garlic.
3. **Add protein** (if using) and sizzle until cooked through.
4. **Add veggies**, flavor crew, and a pinch of salt and pepper. Simmer until tender.
   Pasta still cooking? Just turn off the heat and chill — the skillet's on your schedule.
5. **Add drained pasta** + a splash of pasta water. Toss everything together until glossy.
6. **Finish with cheese**, fresh herbs, and a squeeze of lemon if you're feelin' fancy.

PLAY YOUR WILD CARD

- Want creamy? Stir in a spoonful of cream cheese, yogurt, or goat cheese at the end.
- No fresh herbs? Use dried — just add them earlier so they bloom in the oil.
- Spice it your way — hot to trot or not.
- No pasta fan? No problem — this dish works great with rice, too.

Soba Noodle Alla You

A fusion stir-fry that breaks all the rules — nutty soba noodles (or whatever noodle's loitering in your pantry), garlicky olive oil, Italian-style veggies, and a dash of umami sass. It's part pasta, part stir-fry, and 100% tailored to your taste buds.

Prep Time: 10 min

Cook Time: 10–12 min

Total Time: 20–25 min

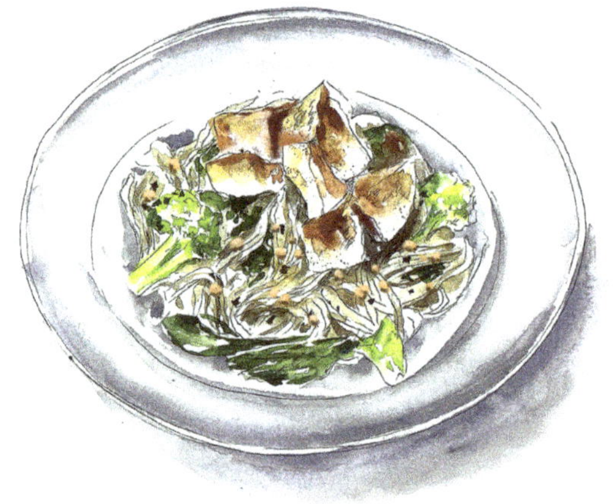

HOW IT'S GONNA GO DOWN

Boil + Stir-Fry

BLOCK PARTY (INGREDIENTS)

This makes one sassy solo portion:

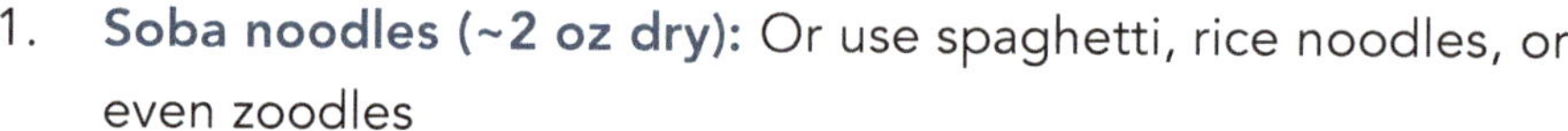

1. **Soba noodles (~2 oz dry):** Or use spaghetti, rice noodles, or even zoodles
2. **Veggies to vibe with (~1–1½ cups total):** Broccoli, zucchini, mushrooms, cherry tomatoes, spinach
3. **Oil (~1 tbsp):** Olive oil or sesame oil

Sauce Combo:

- 1 tsp soy sauce or tamari
- 1 tsp balsamic vinegar
- ½ tsp chili flakes or chili crisp
- Zest of ½ lemon or lime

> *"Italy meets Tokyo in this hot little skillet — and somehow, the flavors just click."*

CALL IN YOUR POWER PLAYERS (~4 oz)

- Shrimp, tofu, or shredded chicken
- Tempeh, edamame, or Italian sausage (yep — it works!)

ASSEMBLE YOUR FLAVOR CREW

- **Italiano Umami:** Garlic, basil, balsamic, spinach
  Top with: shaved Parmesan + chili oil
- **Sesame Street Food:** Toasted sesame, scallions, chili flakes, soy sauce. *Top with:* sesame seeds + lime wedge
- **Garden Groove:** Zucchini, thyme, cherry tomatoes, white beans
  Drizzle with: herby olive oil + lemon zest

HERE'S THE GAME PLAN – BOIL, TOSS, FUSE

1. **Cook soba noodles** according to package directions. Drain and rinse under cold water to stop the cooking and keep them springy.
2. **In a skillet, heat oil and sauté your protein** and flavor crew picks until just cooked, then let the veggies join the sizzle until tender.
3. **Add cooked noodles** and your sauce combo. Toss until everything's well-coated and glossy.
4. **Adjust seasoning**, sprinkle on your favorite toppings, and serve hot in a deep bowl with chopsticks or a fork (no judgment).

PLAY YOUR WILD CARD

- Want it spicy? Add chili garlic sauce or a dab of gochujang.
- Want it creamy? Stir in a spoonful of tahini or cashew cream.
- This dish is all about contrast — warm + cool, savory + zippy, pasta + noodle vibes. Let it play out your way.

Lemony Snickerdish

A cozy, brothy bowl kissed with lemon, herbs, and whatever protein you're vibing with. It's light enough to refresh you, hearty enough to fill you, and easy enough to earn a regular spot in your solo dinner rotation.

Prep Time: 10 min

Cook Time: 15–20 min

Total Time: 25–30 min

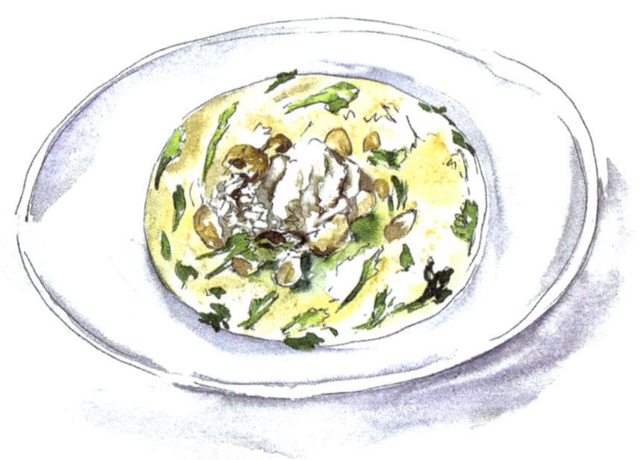

HOW IT'S GONNA GO DOWN

Stovetop Simmer

BLOCK PARTY (INGREDIENTS)

Makes one big bowl of snickerdish.

1. **Chickpeas (~½ can)**
2. **Veggies to vibe with (~½ cup):** Spinach, kale, celery, zucchini, bok choy
3. **Aromatics:** ~1 tsp minced garlic, ¼ small onion or shallot (finely chopped)
4. **Broth (~1½ cups):** Veggie or chicken
5. **Grain (optional, ~¼ cup cooked):** Orzo, small pasta, or rice
6. **Acid:** Juice + zest of ¼ lemon

CALL IN YOUR POWER PLAYERS (Optional)

Chickpeas are the star, but feel free to sub in:

- Beans or lentils (cooked or canned)
- Diced rotisserie chicken
- Seasoned sausage (pre-cooked or ready to eat)
- Tofu

"Plant-powered, meat-friendly — you do you."

ASSEMBLE YOUR FLAVOR CREW

- **Mediterranean Bright:** Lemon zest, oregano, garlic, black pepper
  Top with: crumbled feta + chopped parsley
- **Light & Herby:** Thyme, dill, bay leaf
  Top with: scallions or a swirl of yogurt/sour cream
- **Zesty & Bold:** Cumin, paprika, chili flakes
  Top with: olive oil drizzle + fresh mint

HERE'S THE GAME PLAN – SIZZLE, SIMMER, ZEST

1. **Sauté aromatics** in a splash of olive oil (2–3 minutes).
2. **Add broth**, chickpeas, protein (if using), grains, flavor crew and firm veggies like celery or zucchini. Simmer ~10–12 minutes.
3. **Stir in leafy greens** and lemon juice + zest. Let simmer another 2–3 minutes.
4. **Taste, adjust seasoning**, and top with fresh herbs, crumbled cheese, or a creamy swirl.

PLAY YOUR WILD CARD

- Want it creamier? Mash a few chickpeas with a fork to thicken the broth.
- Use pre-cooked or frozen grains to save time.
- Add a poached or fried egg on top for bonus flair.

Fire & Lime Affair

A spicy, brothy noodle bowl with bold Latin-Asian fusion vibes. Packed with chili, lime, garlic, and noodles, this dish clears your head, warms your soul, and brings the heat — with just enough lime to keep it dangerously refreshing. Now that's an affair worth slurping.

Prep Time: 10 min

Cook Time: 15–20 min

Total Time: 25–30 min

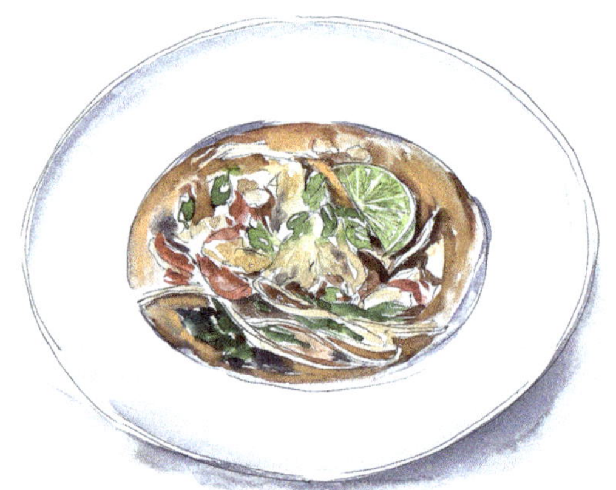

HOW IT'S GONNA GO DOWN

Stovetop Simmer

BLOCK PARTY (INGREDIENTS)

One big slurp-worthy bowl.

1. **Noodles (~2 oz dry):** Rice noodles, soba, or spaghetti
2. **Veggies to vibe with (~1 cup chopped):** Corn, bell pepper, spinach, tomato, scallions
3. **Aromatics:** ~1 tsp each: garlic & ginger + a pinch of chili flakes or fresh chili
4. **Broth (~1½–2 cups):** Veggie, chicken, or miso broth
5. **Sauce boosters:** 1 tsp soy sauce or tamari, ½ tsp hot sauce or chili garlic sauce, and a squeeze of lime to finish

CALL IN YOUR POWER PLAYERS (~4 oz)

- Chicken or pork
- Tofu cubes or edamame
- Shrimp
- Or skip it and let the noodles + broth shine

ASSEMBLE YOUR FLAVOR CREW

- **Spicy Lime:** Chili garlic sauce, lime juice, scallions
  Top with: avocado slices + cilantro
- **Ginger Heat:** Grated ginger, sesame oil, crushed red pepper
  Top with: sriracha + sesame seeds
- **Latin Street Bowl:** Cumin, smoked paprika, corn, tomato
  Top with: crushed tortilla chips + fresh lime

HERE'S THE GAME PLAN – SIZZLE, SIMMER, SLURP

1. **Cook noodles** according to package directions. Drain and set aside.
2. **In the same pot,** heat a splash of oil and cook your protein (if using). Remove and set aside.
3. **Still in the same pot** (to keep dishes to a minimum), **sizzle aromatics** for 1–2 minutes.
4. **Add broth**, sauce boosters (hold the lime), veggies, and your flavor crew. Simmer 7–10 minutes.
5. **Stir in lime juice**. Add cooked noodles and protein.
6. **Heat it all through, give it a taste, tweak** if needed, then top and slurp away.

PLAY YOUR WILD CARD

- Add a soft-boiled egg on top for extra richness.
- Use leftover rotisserie chicken or pre-cooked tofu to save time.
- Want creamy? Stir in a splash of coconut milk or a dollop of yogurt.

Comfort in a Cup (or Bowl)

A velvety veggie soup that's creamy(ish) without the cream, easy to customize, and made for swirling in something bold — yogurt, pesto, chili oil... you do you. Blender optional, flavor mandatory — this one's for solo sippers with serious style.

Prep Time: 10 min

Cook Time: 15–20 min

Total Time: 25–30 min

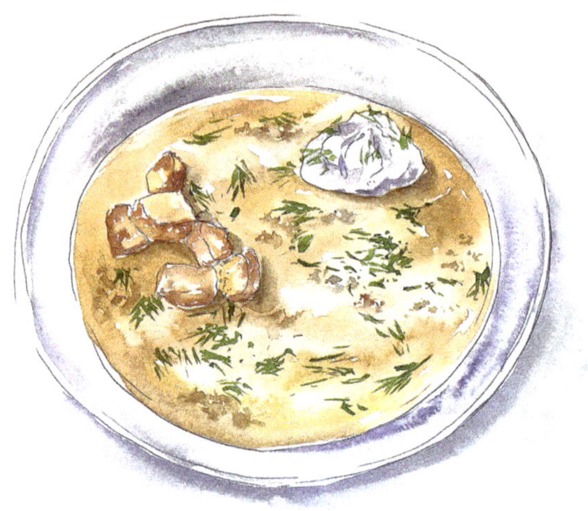

HOW IT'S GONNA GO DOWN

Stovetop Simmer (+ optional blending)

BLOCK PARTY (INGREDIENTS)

Makes one luxurious bowl.

1. **Veggies to vibe with (~1½ cups chopped):** Carrots, cauliflower, broccoli, sweet potato, or a mix
2. **Aromatics:** ~1–2 tsp total of chopped garlic, onion, or shallot
3. **Broth (~1½ cups):** Veggie, chicken or miso
4. **Creamy add-in (optional):** 1–2 tbsp plain yogurt, coconut milk, or cream cheese

CALL IN YOUR POWER PLAYERS (Optional)

- White beans (blended in)
- Shredded chicken (stirred in post-blend)
- Tofu crumbles or tempeh cubes (as a savory topper)

"Or leave it light and let the veggies shine — you're the boss here."

ASSEMBLE YOUR FLAVOR CREW

- **Carrot-Ginger Dream:** Grated ginger, cumin, garlic
  Top with: coconut swirl + chili crisp
- **Broccoli Herb Cream:** Thyme, dill, lemon zest
  Top with: Greek yogurt + croutons
- **Cozy Sweet Potato:** Cinnamon, smoked paprika, cayenne
  Top with: toasted seeds + maple or hot sauce drizzle

HERE'S THE GAME PLAN – SIZZLE, SIMMER, SWIRL

1. **In a small pot, sauté** aromatics in oil (2–3 minutes).
2. **Add chopped veggies**, flavor crew, and broth. Bring to a boil, then simmer 12–15 minutes until veggies are fork-tender.
3. **Blend until smooth** (with immersion blender or in batches).
4. **Return to pot**, stir in your creamy add-in, and season to taste.
5. **Swirl in toppings** and serve warm.

PLAY YOUR WILD CARD

- No blender? Mash it rustic-style with a fork or potato masher.
- Add crunch: roasted chickpeas, croutons, or seed sprinkle.
- Want it chilled in summer? Totally works — just top with fresh herbs and keep it cool.

Tabbouleh, Your Way

A bright, herby grain salad that's refreshing, satisfying, and totally open to interpretation. Traditionally made with bulgur, parsley, mint, lemon, and tomato — but around here, we remix it based on what's in the fridge. It's the kind of dish that says "I've got this" without even turning on the stove.

Prep Time: 10–15 min (plus grain cooking time if needed)

Cook Time: 0–10 min (depending on grain)

Total Time: 15–25 min

HOW IT'S GONNA GO DOWN

No-Cook (with pre-cooked grain) or Quick Simmer

BLOCK PARTY (INGREDIENTS) — For One Serving

1. **Grain (~¼ cup dry = ~½ cup cooked):** Traditional: bulgur
   Also works: quinoa, couscous, farro, rice, or cauliflower rice
2. **Veggies to vibe with (~1 cup):** Tomato, cucumber, scallions, or red onion. Optional: bell pepper, radish, shredded carrot
3. **Fresh herbs (~½ cup total):** Parsley (must-have), mint (highly recommended), dill, basil. cilantro (optional extras)
4. **Acid + oil:** Juice of ½ lemon or lime + 1–2 tbsp olive oil
5. **Aromatics:** Salt, pepper, garlic (optional)

CALL IN YOUR POWER PLAYERS (~½ cup or so)

- Crumbled feta or goat cheese
- Chickpeas or white beans
- Diced avocado
- Leftover grilled chicken or shrimp

"Or just keep it pure and herb-powered — you can't go wrong."

ASSEMBLE YOUR FLAVOR CREW

- **Traditional Style:** Bulgur + parsley + mint + tomato + cucumber + lemon + olive oil
  No feta, no fluff — just classic simplicity
- **Mediterranean Remix:** Quinoa + parsley + dill + feta + kalamata olives + red onion + lemon + olive oil
- **Southwest Vibe:** Couscous + cilantro + corn + black beans + avocado + lime juice + chili flakes
- **Clean Green Crunch:** Cauliflower rice + mint + cucumber + pumpkin seeds + tahini drizzle

HERE'S THE GAME PLAN – CHOP, FLUFF, CHILL

1. If needed, **cook and cool your grain** of choice.
2. **Chop herbs and veggies finely.**
3. **Toss everything together** in a bowl with lemon juice, olive oil, salt, and pepper.
4. **Let sit for 10–15 minutes** if you can — the flavor only gets better.
5. **Serve as-is**, on a bed of greens, or wrapped in lettuce or pita.

PLAY YOUR WILD CARD

- Great for meal prep: Double the grain + herbs and remix each day.
- Add protein: Turn it into a full meal or serve as a side with grilled dishes.
- No waste hero: Rescue herbs on the verge of wilting — just chop and toss.

In a Pickle (and Loving It)

This isn't your average "sad solo salad." It's got zing, it's got bite, and it's got just enough creamy swagger to keep things smooth. With crisp lettuce, juicy veggies, chopped pickles, and a creamy-tangy dressing that throws shade at store-bought bottles, this bowl is your new go-to when you want something quick, crunchy, and unapologetically bold.

Prep Time: 10–15 min

Cook Time: 5–10 min (if cooking protein)

Total Time: 15–20 min

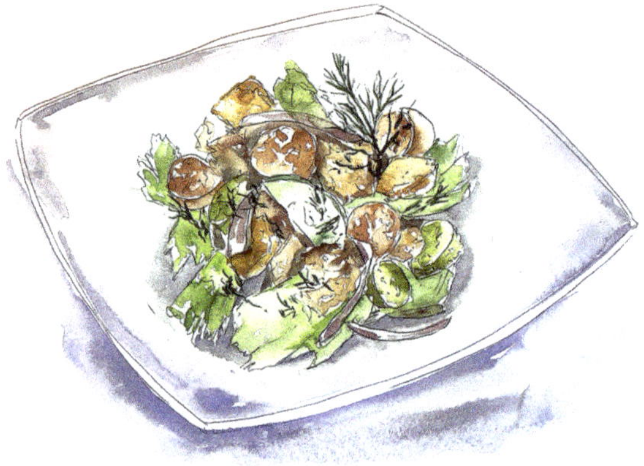

HOW IT'S GONNA GO DOWN

Quick Sauté + Toss

BLOCK PARTY (INGREDIENTS)

Build your base with ~2 cups total for a solo-sized bowl.

1. **Crunchy stuff:** Chopped romaine, shredded iceberg, or mixed greens
2. **Juicy bits:** Halved cherry tomatoes, diced cucumber
3. **Zingy extras:** Chopped dill pickles, sliced red onion
4. **Creamy-Tangy Dressing (~2–3 tbsp total):**
   ~1 tbsp mayo, ~1 tsp each of ketchup, white wine vinegar, and pickle juice, ~½ tsp mustard, salt & pepper to taste

CALL IN YOUR POWER PLAYERS (~4 oz)

- Sautéed ground beef, turkey, or chicken
- Plant-based crumbles
- Chickpeas or white beans (for no-cook ease)
- Chopped hard-boiled egg
- Canned tuna

ASSEMBLE YOUR FLAVOR CREW

- **Fresh & Bright:** Fresh dill, chives, or scallions
- **Savory & Mild:** Paprika, black pepper
- **Cheesy & Bold:** Crumbled feta, goat cheese, or your favorite shredded blend

HERE'S THE GAME PLAN – COOK, CHOP, SAUCE IT UP

1. **In a skillet, cook your protein** (if using) in a splash of oil with salt & pepper. Set aside.
2. **Mix all dressing ingredients** in a small bowl or jar. Taste and tweak as needed.
3. **Place chopped lettuce** and veggies into a bowl.
4. **Drizzle dressing** over and toss to coat evenly.
5. **Top with protein** (warm or chilled), sprinkle with your flavor crew, and finish with any extras — cheese, herbs, fresh cracked pepper, or whatever you're feeling.

PLAY YOUR WILD CARD

- Craving crunch? Add croutons, toasted seeds, or potato sticks (seriously).
- No pickle juice? Sub with more vinegar and a dash of sugar.
- Spice it up with a dash of hot sauce or cayenne in the dressing.

Bowl'd & Boujee (Fancy, That Is!)

A rainbow of superfoods meets bold, crunchy, juicy goodness — all tossed in a bright, creamy citrus dressing that makes your body and your taste buds do a happy dance. It's nutrient-packed, fridge-friendly, and fully customizable. This bowl isn't just healthy — it's clean-out-the-fridge genius dressed in five-star flair.

Prep Time: 10 min

Cook Time: 15 min

Total Time: 25 min

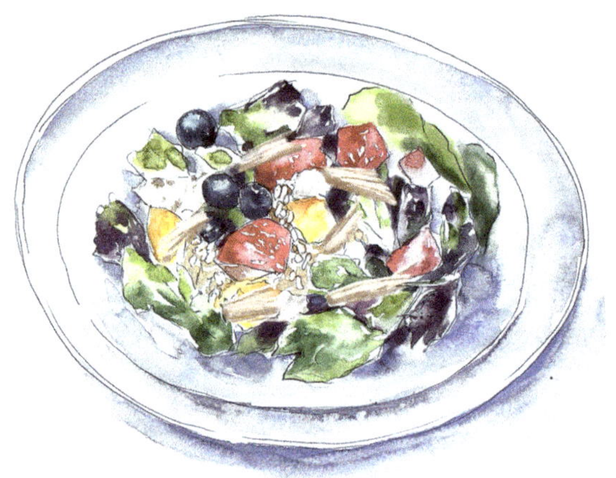

HOW IT'S GONNA GO DOWN

Quick Simmer + No-Cook Assembly

BLOCK PARTY (INGREDIENTS)

Makes one big bowl of boujee bliss.

1. **Grain (~½ cup cooked):** Quinoa, farro, bulgur, or rice
2. **Greens (~1½–2 cups):** Kale, spinach, arugula, or whatever's hanging out in your fridge
3. **Fruity Boost (~½–¾ cup total):** Blueberries, halved grapes, chopped apple or pear, dried cherries or cranberries
4. **Crunch Zone (~¼ cup each):** Sunflower seeds, chopped walnuts, or pumpkin seeds
5. **Cheese (optional, ~¼ cup):** Feta, goat cheese, or Parmesan — crumbled or shredded

CALL IN YOUR POWER PLAYERS (~½ cup or 4–6 oz)

- Cooked edamame, white beans or chickpeas
- Rotisserie chicken or grilled tofu
- Canned tuna or chicken
- Or skip the extras and ride the veggie wave

ASSEMBLE YOUR FLAVOR CREW

- **Citrus-Garlic Creamy Vibe:**
  ~1 tbsp each orange juice + olive oil
  ~1 pinch each minced garlic + sugar
  Salt + pepper to taste
  Shake it up first, then stir in Greek yogurt or sour cream for dreamy creaminess.
- **Zesty Honey-Dijon Vinaigrette:**
  ~2 tbsp olive oil, drizzle of lemon juice
  ~½ tsp each Dijon mustard + honey
  Splash of apple cider vinegar
  Shake it like you mean it. Creamy upgrade? Stir in yogurt or sour cream.

HERE'S THE GAME PLAN – MIX, SHAKE, DEVOUR

1. **Cook your grain and protein** (like edamame) according to package directions.
2. **In a big ol' bowl, toss together** greens, grains, fruit, protein, cheese (if using), and all your crunchy bits.
3. **Shake up dressing** ingredients in a jar until creamy and fully blended.
4. **Pour it over, toss it up, taste and adjust** — then get ready to swoon.

PLAY YOUR WILD CARD

- Add a jammy egg, crispy tofu, or leftover roasted veggies for a glow-up.
- Want even more feel-good vibes? Drizzle with balsamic glaze or a spoon of tahini.
- Got fruit on its last leg? Dice it in — this bowl doesn't judge.

Pasta La Vista, Boring

A fast, flavorful pasta dish that's endlessly remixable — veggie-packed, protein-optional, and ready in the time it takes to boil water. Fry up your faves while the pasta cooks, then bring it all together in one glorious pan. Creamy? Zingy? Herby? You call the vibe.

Prep Time: 5 min

Cook Time: 15 min

Total Time: 20 min

HOW IT'S GONNA GO DOWN

Stovetop Boil + Skillet Sauté + Toss & Heat

BLOCK PARTY (INGREDIENTS)

1. **Pasta (~¾ cup dry / 1½ cups cooked):** Penne, fusilli, spaghetti, linguine (GF if needed)
2. **Veggies to vibe with (~1–1½ cups total):** Choose 1–3 based on the flavor profile:
   - *Earthy & Bold:* Broccoli, radicchio
   - *Green & Bright:* Zucchini, green asparagus, peas, chives
   - *Savory & Smoky:* Eggplant, red onion, cherry tomato
   - *Fresh & Light:* Red onion, spinach, artichokes, fennel
3. **Crunchy Topper (~2–3 tbsp):** Toasted hazelnuts, walnuts, pine nuts, or breadcrumbs
4. **Zing Factor (optional):** Lemon zest or juice, vinegar splash, chili flakes
5. **Cheese (~¼ cup, optional):** Parmesan, goat cheese, feta, or dairy-free shred

CALL IN YOUR POWER PLAYERS (~4–6 oz)

- Crispy chorizo or sausage (meat or plant-based)
- White fish (cubed)
- Chicken or tofu (cubed)
- Cannellini beans or chickpeas

ASSEMBLE YOUR FLAVOR CREW

- **Herby & Bright:** Basil, parsley, chives, lemon zest
- **Savory & Earthy:** Oregano, thyme, smoked paprika
- **Spicy & Bold:** Chili flakes, garlic, lemon juice, sharp cheese

HERE'S THE GAME PLAN – BOIL, SIZZLE, TOSS

1. **Cook pasta** in salted water until al dente. Reserve a splash of pasta water.
2. **While pasta cooks, heat olive oil in a skillet.**
   - If using raw protein (like chicken or fish), sauté it first until nearly cooked through.
   - Then add your veggies and cook until tender.
   - If using pre-cooked protein (like sausage or tofu), add it with the veggies instead.
   - Season everything with salt, pepper, and your flavor crew.
3. **Add drained pasta** to skillet. Toss everything together with reserved pasta water, add cheese if using and toss again until glossy and hot (about 2-3 min).
4. **Top with nuts or breadcrumbs.** Taste and adjust seasoning — now serve and strut.

PLAY YOUR WILD CARD

- Add a spoonful of pesto, tapenade, or sun-dried tomato paste.
- Toss in arugula or spinach at the end for a wilted green touch.
- Craving creamy? Stir in ricotta, Greek yogurt, sour cream, or plain cream cheese. Even a splash of heavy cream or half-and-half brings instant richness to the party.

Ricotta Be Kidding Me

Who says dinner has to be hot, heavy, or complicated? This bold little toast brings the flavor and the flair — creamy herbed ricotta, juicy roasted grapes or blistered cherry tomatoes, and a drizzle of something fabulous. It's the kind of meal that proves "just toast" can totally count as dinner… especially when it's this dressed up. Light, satisfying, and endlessly riffable — this one's your solo evening upgrade, no stove stress required.

Prep Time: 10 min

Cook Time: 10–15 min (optional, if roasting grapes or tomatoes)

Total Time: 10–20 min

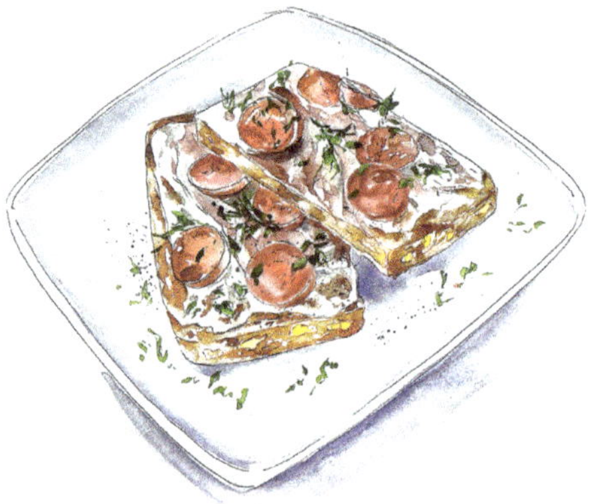

HOW IT'S GONNA GO DOWN

No-Cook or Quick Roast + Toast Assembly

BLOCK PARTY (INGREDIENTS)

Makes one fabulous toast.

1. **Bread (1 thick slice):** Sourdough, multigrain, or any crusty slice you love
2. **Ricotta (~¼-½ cup):** Regular or whipped — or check the *Wild Card* section for tasty swaps
3. **Herbs (~1 tbsp chopped):** Basil, chives, parsley, thyme — your pick
4. **Toppings (~¼–⅓ cup):** Roasted grapes, cherry tomatoes, or sautéed mushrooms - see flavor crew for different combos
5. **Finishers (to taste):** Olive oil, balsamic glaze, flaky salt, cracked pepper, lemon zest

CALL IN YOUR POWER PLAYERS (~2–4 oz, optional)

- Sliced prosciutto
- Crumbled bacon
- Smoked salmon
- White beans or chickpeas (smashed with olive oil + lemon)

ASSEMBLE YOUR FLAVOR CREW

- **Sweet & Herby:** Thyme, basil, roasted grapes, balsamic glaze
- **Savory Umami:** Garlic oil, sautéed mushrooms, cracked pepper
- **Zesty Fresh:** Lemon zest, chives, cherry tomatoes, olive oil drizzle

HERE'S THE GAME PLAN – TOAST, SPREAD, STACK

1. **Toast your bread** until golden and crisp.
2. **If roasting grapes or tomatoes:** toss with a drizzle of olive oil + pinch of salt, roast at 400°F (200°C) for 10–15 minutes.
3. **Mix ricotta** with your chopped herbs and a pinch of salt and pepper.
4. **Spread the herbed ricotta** generously over the toast.
5. **Add your toppings** (warm or chilled), drizzle with balsamic or olive oil, and finish with flaky salt or lemon zest, or a little magic from your flavor crew.
6. **Serve warm** or room temp — with a simple side salad if you're feelin' a little extra.

PLAY YOUR WILD CARD

- No ricotta? Swap in creamy goat cheese, whipped cream cheese, or even hummus.
- Craving different flavors? Try roasted red peppers, caramelized onions, or whatever your heart desires.
- Add a crunch: Top with toasted pine nuts, chopped walnuts, or a sprinkle of crispy breadcrumbs.

Queso Amor

A golden, crispy tortilla enveloping melty cheese and your choice of flavorful fillings—this quesadilla is the ultimate quick-fix dinner. Ready in under 20 minutes, it's perfect for those nights when you crave something comforting without the fuss.

Prep Time: 5–10 min

Cook Time: 5–10 min

Total Time: 10–20 min

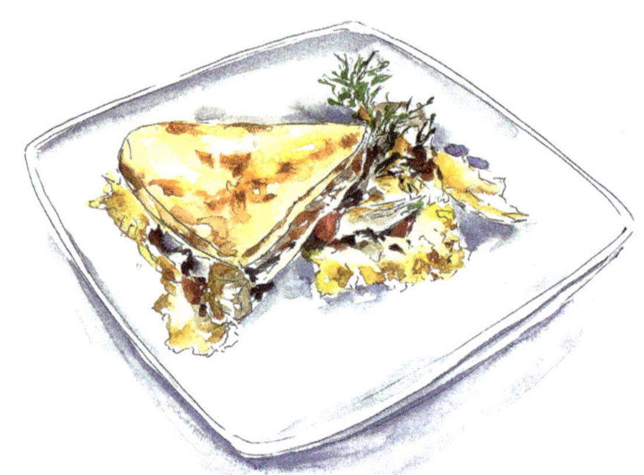

HOW IT'S GONNA GO DOWN

Stovetop Sizzle + Fold & Crisp

BLOCK PARTY (INGREDIENTS)

Serves 1 hungry human

1. **Tortilla:** 1 large flour tortilla (8–10 inches, burrito size)
2. **Veggies to vibe with (~¼–½ cup):** Finely chopped bell peppers, onions, mushrooms, spinach, corn, or any leftovers
3. **Aromatics (~½ tsp each):** Garlic, scallions, or jalapeños (optional)
4. **Cheese (~½ cup):** Cheddar, Monterey Jack, mozzarella, or a blend (dairy-free works, too)
5. **Oil or Butter:** For crisping the tortilla

CALL IN YOUR POWER PLAYERS (~4 oz)

- ➟ Cooked chicken, steak, or shrimp
- ➟ Black beans or pinto beans
- ➟ Sautéed tofu or tempeh
- ➟ Leftover roasted vegetables

ASSEMBLE YOUR FLAVOR CREW

- **Classic:** Cumin, chili powder, garlic powder
- **Herby:** Fresh cilantro, parsley, or chives
- **Spicy:** Hot sauce, red pepper flakes, or chipotle powder

HERE'S THE GAME PLAN – FILL, FOLD, SIZZLE

1. **Prep the Filling:** Sauté veggies and aromatics (like garlic or scallions) in a skillet with a bit of oil until tender. Add your chosen protein and flavor crew. Stir until everything's heated through and flavorful. Remove from skillet and set aside.
2. **Assemble the Quesadilla:** Wipe the skillet clean and place it over medium heat. Place the tortilla in the skillet, sprinkle half the cheese over one side (you'll be folding it like a taco). Add the filling, then top with the remaining cheese.
3. **Cook:** Fold the tortilla over the filling to create a half-moon shape. Cook for 2–3 minutes on each side, pressing down gently, until both sides are golden and cheese is melted.
4. **Serve:** Transfer to a cutting board, let it sit for a minute (it helps everything stay together, then slice into wedges. Serve with your favorite dips like salsa, guacamole, or sour cream.

PLAY YOUR WILD CARD

- Out of Tortillas? Use a flatbread — or go low-carb with a large lettuce leaf wrap.
- Extra Crunch: Add crushed tortilla chips inside before cooking.
- Breakfast Twist: Fill with scrambled eggs, cheese, and breakfast sausage for a morning delight.

Fry Me to the Moon

A fast, fiery stir-fry that's all about flavor, flexibility, and frying with flair. Toss in what you've got, sauce it like you mean it, and prepare for takeoff. This one's got late-night cravings and solo kitchen dancing written all over it.

Prep Time: 10–15 min

Cook Time: 10–15 min

Total Time: 20–30 min

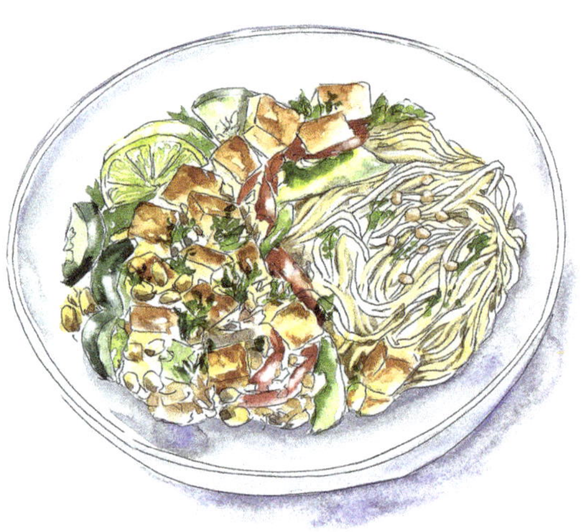

HOW IT'S GONNA GO DOWN

Stovetop Sizzle + Stir-Fry Blitz

BLOCK PARTY (Ingredients)

Choose your base and build your bowl.

1. **Veggies to vibe with (~1½–2 cups):** Bell pepper strips, snap peas or green beans, broccoli florets, carrot ribbons, mushrooms, baby corn or water chestnuts, shredded cabbage or kale, zucchini or bok choy
2. **Toppings (optional):** Green onion (for that fancy finish)
3. **Grain Option (~1 cup cooked, optional):** Rice, rice noodles, quinoa, or cauliflower rice — if you want to bulk it up or soak up that saucy goodness

CALL IN YOUR POWER PLAYERS (~4–6 oz)

Pick what you've got or what you're craving:

- Chicken or turkey breast (thinly sliced)
- Shrimp or scallops
- Tofu or tempeh (cubed)
- Eggs (scrambled right in)
- Leftover steak or pork (thin slices)

ASSEMBLE YOUR FLAVOR CREW – PICK A SAUCE VIBE

- **Sweet Chili Lime**
  ~ 1 tbsp sweet chili sauce, 1 tsp lime juice, 1 tsp soy or tamari, pinch of red pepper flakes (optional)
- **Ginger-Sesame Zing**
  ~ 1 tbsp soy or tamari, 1 tsp sesame oil, ½ tsp grated fresh ginger, dash of rice vinegar
- **Peanut Umami Bomb**
  ~ 1 tbsp peanut butter, 1 tsp soy or tamari, splash of warm water to thin, dash of sriracha or chili crisp

HERE'S THE GAME PLAN – CHOP, SIZZLE, SAUCE, SOAR

1. **Chop + Prep** – Slice your veggies and protein. Mix your sauce in a small bowl.
2. **Sizzle That Protein** – Heat oil in a large skillet or wok. Cook it golden, cook it through, then give it a break on the sidelines.
3. **Veggie Action** – In the same skillet, add a splash of oil if the pan is dry and stir-fry veggies for 4–6 minutes until crisp-tender.
4. **Sauce + Toss** – Add the protein back in. Pour sauce over everything and stir until all that goodness is glossy and sauced to perfection.
5. **Plate Up** – Serve over your chosen grain or straight from the pan — no judgment.

PLAY YOUR WILD CARD

- Swap in frozen stir-fry veggies if you're short on fresh.
- Add cashews or sesame seeds for crunch.
- Going for a pop of freshness? Top with fresh cilantro or basil.
- Pantry running low? Mix soy sauce + hot sauce + honey and call it a day.

Board Out Of My Mind

No stove. No stress. Just a perfectly balanced board of nibbles, dips, and little delights that totally counts as dinner. Whether you're grazing, multitasking, or living your best snack-cuterie life— this one's proof that dinner doesn't have to be hot to be hot.

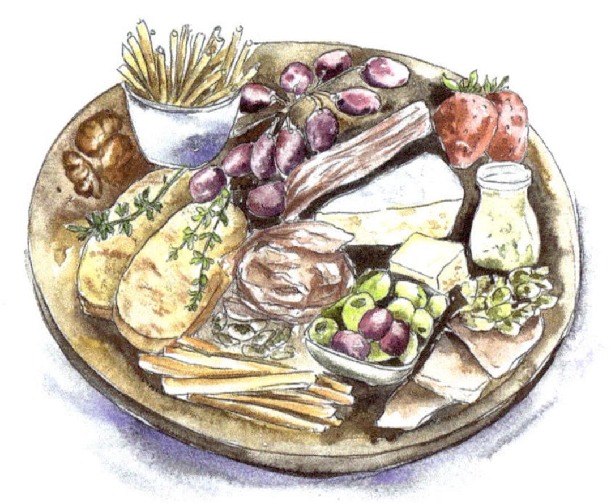

Prep Time: 5–10 min

Cook Time: 0 min

Total Time: 5–10 min

HOW IT'S GONNA GO DOWN

No-Cook Assembly

BUILD YOUR BOARD – PICK 1–2 FROM EACH SECTION

1. **Protein Power (~4–6 oz total):**
   Hard-boiled egg
   Deli turkey or chicken
   Smoked salmon
   Hummus or bean dip
   Cheese (cubed or sliced)
   Leftover grilled tofu or tempeh
2. **Crunchy Stuff (~½–1 cup):**
   Crackers, pita chips, pretzels
   Roasted chickpeas or nuts
   Seeded flatbread or tortilla chips
3. **Color & Crunch (~1 cup):**
   Baby carrots, cucumber slices, bell pepper strips
   Cherry tomatoes, sugar snap peas
   Pickles or olives (yes, they count)

4. **Something Juicy (~½ cup):**
   Grapes, apple slices, berries, orange wedges
   Dried fruit like apricots or dates

5. **Saucy Situation (1–2 tbsp):**
   Hummus, tzatziki, ranch, mustard, nut butter
   Yes, even that lonely jar of fig jam or hot honey hiding in the back of your fridge.

CHOOSE YOUR VIBE

- **Chill & Balanced**: Turkey, hummus, cucumbers, crackers, apple slices, peanut butter
- **Euro Vibes**: Cheddar, salami, grapes, seeded crisps, mustard, olives
- **Plant-Powered**: Tofu, roasted chickpeas, carrots, grapes, tahini dip, dark chocolate square
- **Latin-Inspired**: Sliced chicken, tortilla chips, black bean dip, cherry tomatoes, mango

ASSEMBLE YOUR FLAVOR CREW

This one's all about little add-ons:

- Sprinkle chili-lime seasoning on fruit
- Drizzle hot honey on cheese or crackers
- Add flaky sea salt to sliced tomato or cucumber

PLAY YOUR WILD CARD

- Arrange it on a cute plate or cutting board — you deserve the full aesthetic.
- This is dinner. Full stop. No oven, no judgment.
- Bonus points for pairing it with a great show, a chill playlist, or a quiet moment.

Solutions for When You'd Rather Snack Than Sauté

When even building a snack board feels like too much.

If "assembling a board" sounds like work and turning on the stove is a firm heck no — but your taste buds still want something real, satisfying, and slightly fabulous — here are a few lazy-day combos that bring big flavor with zero heat and barely any effort.

Just grab what you've got, mix and match, and call it dinner. *(No shame. All snack game.)*

Snack Plate Win

Fresh crunchy veggies or leftover roasted ones + store-bought hummus + a boiled egg
= Dip, dunk, devour — dinner's done.

Wrap It & Roll

Tuna or chicken salad + avocado + tortilla or lettuce leaves
= Wrap it and go.

Lazy Day Salad

Canned beans + cherry tomatoes + feta + olive oil + squeeze of lemon
= Fresh, filling, and fork-friendly.

Surprise Snack Bowl

Greek yogurt + chickpeas + lemon + flaky salt
= Creamy, tangy, and unexpectedly awesome.

Deli Stack Hack

Sliced turkey *or any deli meat* + cheese + mustard + pickles
= Layer it, roll it, or eat it straight from the cutting board.

Breakfast-for-Dinner Bowl

Yogurt + fruit + nut butter + granola or seeds
= Sweet, simple, and secretly smart.

Mediterranean Mash-Up

Store-bought tabbouleh or couscous salad + hummus + olives + greens + feta = Toss it in a bowl and drizzle with love (aka olive oil).

Grown-Up PB&J (Kinda)

Whole grain toast or crackers + nut butter + sliced banana or berries + flaky salt = Comfort food with a glow-up.

Pro tip:

Raid your fridge for leftovers, dips, or that last scoop of pesto — and don't underestimate the power of a good drizzle (olive oil, hot honey, you name it).

You're not skipping dinner. You're upgrading chill.

Bonus: Sauce It, Stir It, Drizzle It

Because even a simple dish deserves a little extra.

Let's be real — sometimes all it takes to go from meh to *heck yes* is one bold drizzle. These small-but-mighty sauces are your secret weapons — perfect for bowls, toasts, wraps, roasted veggies, or straight off the spoon (no judgment). You won't need fancy gadgets or chef-school skills. Just a jar, a spoon, and a few pantry staples.

What you'll find here:

- ➡ Small-batch recipes made just for one
- ➡ Quick blends — literally done in minutes
- ➡ No giant bottles gathering dust in the fridge
- ➡ And definitely no mystery goo (lookin' at you, xanthan gum)

These recipes are all real-food flavor boosters — no unpronounceables, no waste, just bold, craveable sauces made for solo cooks who want their meals to *slap* without extra clutter or cost.

So, let's sauce it, stir it, and drizzle it, my friend.

Peanut Sauce, Please!

Creamy, nutty, and just the right amount of sweet-meets-salty — this sauce brings big flavor with zero fuss. Use it on stir-fries, bowls, wraps, or anything that needs a quick upgrade from boring to boujee.

What You'll Need:

⅓ cup creamy peanut butter

½ tsp freshly minced ginger *or* ¼ tsp ground ginger

1 tbsp maple syrup

2 tbsp low-sodium soy sauce

1 tsp rice wine vinegar or lemon juice

½ tsp sesame seeds

¼ tsp crushed red pepper flakes *(optional)*

2–4 tbsp hot water *(to thin as needed)*

Pro tip:
Try it as a dip for roasted sweet potatoes or a spread on your next wrap — you won't regret it.

What You'll Do:

Stir or whisk everything together in a bowl or jar until smooth and creamy. Add hot water a spoonful at a time until you reach your dream consistency — thick enough to coat, thin enough to drizzle. Taste and tweak to match your vibe.

Yield:

About ½ cup of sauce (enough for 2–3 solo meals or one flavor-loaded dinner-for-two— should you happen to have a guest)

Fridge Life:

Store in an airtight container in the fridge for up to **5 days**. The sauce may thicken — just stir in a splash of hot water or a bit of lime juice to loosen it up.

Pesto Party for One

A punchy, herby spread that's good on pasta, toast, wraps, bowls — and even scrambled eggs. This version is small-batch, no special equipment needed, and totally remixable depending on your herbs, nuts, or mood.

What You'll Need:

1 packed cup fresh herbs *(basil, parsley, arugula, cilantro — or a mix)*

1 small garlic clove *(or half a large one)*

2 tbsp toasted nuts or seeds *(pine nuts, walnuts, almonds, sunflower seeds — you do you)*

2 tbsp grated Parmesan or nutritional yeast *(optional)*

Juice of ¼ lemon

2–3 tbsp olive oil *(plus more as needed to loosen)*

Pinch of salt + pepper to taste

Pro tip:
Mix with yogurt or sour cream for a quick pesto dip. Or swirl it into soup — you fanc.

What You'll Do:

Finely chop the garlic and herbs. Add nuts and chop everything together until it's as smooth or rustic as you like. Stir in lemon juice, Parmesan (if using), and olive oil until it becomes a spoonable paste. Taste, adjust, and swirl on everything.

Yield:

About ⅓–½ cup — enough for 1–2 generous pasta bowls or a few flavor-packed drizzles over the week.

Fridge Life: Store in an airtight jar for **3–4 days**. Cover with a thin layer of olive oil on top to keep it fresh.

Freezer Tip: Freeze extra in small portions (ice cube trays work great!) and thaw just what you need.

So Low Hummus

This small-batch hummus is creamy, zippy, and ready in minutes — no giant blender required. It's great as a dip, a spread, or a last-minute "I'm-too-hungry-to-cook" meal base. Customize it with whatever you've got and swirl it like you're running a mezze bar.

What You'll Need:

½ can chickpeas *(drained + rinsed)*
1 tbsp tahini *(or skip it and use olive oil only)*
Juice of ½ lemon
1 small garlic clove *(or use a pinch of garlic powder if you're feeling lazy)*
1½–2 tbsp olive oil
Pinch of salt
1–3 tbsp water, as needed to thin

What You'll Do:

Mash chickpeas with a fork or blend in a mini food processor. Add tahini, lemon, garlic, olive oil, and a splash of water. Stir or blend until creamy. Adjust thickness with more water, and season to taste.

Yield:

About ½ cup — just enough to satisfy, not enough to overwhelm.

Fridge Life:

Store in an airtight container for **up to 5 days**.

Flavor Swaps (a.k.a. Wild Cards):

Add cumin, smoked paprika, or chili flakes for a little heat.
Stir in roasted red pepper or sun-dried tomatoes.
Top with a drizzle of olive oil + toasted seeds or herbs.

Pro tip:
If you love hummus but hate garlic breath, roast the garlic first — or skip it and no one will know but you.

Sriracha Mayo (or Yogurt)

Creamy, spicy, and done in 30 seconds — this one's perfect on wraps, bowls, roasted veggies, or anything that needs a little heat and hug.

What You'll Need:

2 tbsp mayo *or* plain yogurt

1–2 tsp sriracha *(adjust to your spice mood)*

Squeeze of lime juice *(optional, but yum)*

Pinch of garlic powder or smoked paprika *(optional)*

What You'll Do:
Mix it all in a small bowl or jar until smooth. Taste and tweak. That's it.

Yield:
About 2–3 tablespoons — enough for 1–2 meals.

Fridge Life:
Up to **5 days** in a sealed container. Stir before using if it separates.

Chipotle Mayo (or Yogurt)

Smoky, creamy, and bold — this one's a flavor bomb for tacos, bowls, or roasted sweet potatoes.

What You'll Need:

2 tbsp mayo *or* plain yogurt

1 tsp chipotle hot sauce

Pinch of garlic powder

Dash of lime juice or vinegar *(optional)*

What You'll Do:

Stir everything together in a jar or bowl.
Taste and add more adobo for heat,
more lime for tang.

Yield:

About 2–3 tablespoons

Fridge Life:

Lasts **4–5 days** sealed. A little goes a long way, so small batch = smart.

Pro tip:
Make a neutral base (just mayo + lime) and divide it — spice up one half with sriracha, the other with chipotle. Boom, two sauces in one move.

Quick Drizzles & Dollops

(A few bold little sauces for when your bowl needs a boost)

Avocado Crema: Mash ½ avocado with 1 tbsp plain yogurt or sour cream + a squeeze of lime + pinch of salt. (*Lasts 1–2 days in the fridge. Best fresh.*)

Yogurt-Tahini: Mix 1 tbsp tahini + 2 tbsp yogurt + splash of lemon juice + pinch of garlic powder. (*Fridge life: 3 days.*)

Soy-Ginger Drizzle: 1 tbsp soy sauce + ½ tsp sesame oil + grated ginger + splash of rice vinegar. (*Great on bowls or stir-fries. Lasts 3–4 days.*)

Lime Vinaigrette: 2 tbsp olive oil + juice of ½ lime + ½ tsp honey + pinch of salt & pepper. Shake it up. (*Fridge life: 4–5 days.*)

Simple Vinaigrette: 2 tbsp olive oil + 1 tbsp vinegar (balsamic, red wine, or apple cider) + ½ tsp Dijon mustard + pinch of salt & pepper.

Whisk or shake in a jar until blended. *Too puckery? Add a teensy drizzle of honey or a pinch of sugar to mellow things out. Your vinaigrette, your rules.* (*Fridge life: 5 days. Just shake before using.*)

The End? Nah. Just the Delicious Beginning

While this might be the last page of this cookbook, it's *definitely* not the end of your flavor journey. In fact, this is where things really start to get fun.

By now, you've seen how each dish in here can flex with your mood, your fridge, or your cravings. So, what's next? You keep going — that's what. Try a dish you loved with a new Power Player. Mix up your Flavor Crew. Swap in different grains or veggies from your latest grocery haul (or leftovers).

You've already got the formula:

Pick your cooking method

Gather your Block Party ingredients

Call in your Power Players

Assemble your Flavor Crew

And get that skillet sizzling

This book has a solid month of recipes — but with just a few swaps, you've got enough combos to last you *three or four months*. No burnout. No boredom. Just food that fits your life — and your flavor.

And maybe most important of all: this isn't only about cooking. It's about choosing yourself. You're worth the effort it takes to make a flavorful, satisfying meal — even (and especially) when it's just for you.

So, keep going. Keep playing. Keep feeding yourself like you matter.

Because you absolutely do.

A Little Flavor Favor

If this book has added a little more joy, ease, or flavor to your solo kitchen life — would you help me pass the magic on?

Whether you're feeling more confident in the kitchen, getting creative with what's in your fridge, or simply enjoying dinner more these days… I'd be so grateful if you shared the love.

A quick, honest review on Amazon (or wherever you picked up this book!) helps other solo cooks find their way to flavor — and gives this little book a longer life. If you think five stars are earned, I'd be extra grateful.

As a thank-you, I've got something just for you —
The Dinner for One Toolkit: your all-in-one support system for solo kitchen wins.
Inside, you'll find:

A 4-week solo meal plan — take the guesswork out of dinner and keep things fresh

Flexible shopping lists — tailored for solo cooking, so nothing goes to waste

Smart pantry setup tips — stock your kitchen with ease, not overload

A printable Flavor Journal page — track your swaps, wins, and flavor discoveries…plus more ways to keep solo cooking simple, fun, and full of flavor.

Visit **www.rockthekitchen.net/dinnerforonetoolkit** or scan the QR code below to grab your bonus bundle.

And hey — I'd love to see what you're cooking!

Tag me on Instagram @kerstindecook using **#DinnerForOneCookbook** so I can cheer you on, celebrate your solo wins, and maybe even share your plate with our flavor-loving crew.

OR join our growing kitchen-loving crew on Facebook here: https://bit.ly/join-rockthekitchen — where flavor, confidence, and creativity are always on the menu. Whether it's a cozy one-pan dinner, a bold bowl remix, or a total flavor experiment — I'm here for it.

Thanks for being part of this one-pan, one-plate, one-happy-belly adventure.

Let's keep rocking the kitchen, my friend.

With flavor and gratitude,

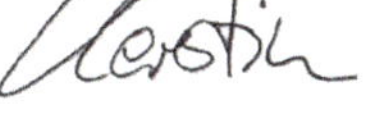

The Menu: Dished Out

(alphabetized)

A full spread of solo stunners — find your flavor, get a quick peek, and dig into whatever calls your name.

Bake It Till You Make It – Roasty, toasty, and smugly delicious. 66

Bangkok in a Pan – A flavor trip to Thailand, minus the jet lag. 62

Balls of Glory – Juicy little flavor bombs with veggie backup. 44

Board Out Of My Mind – Dinner? Barely. Delicious? Absolutely. 108

Bowl'd & Boujee – Superfood star treatment, à la carte. 98

Comfort in a Cup (or Bowl) – Sip, slurp, savor, repeat. 92

Crust Me, It's Good – Golden, gooey, and gone in 60 seconds. 80

Curry Me Home – Creamy, cozy, and spoon-lickin' good. 40

Egg-cellent for One – A solo frittata adventure—easy, breezy, and egg-stra tasty. 46

Egg-cuse Me, Dinner? – Bold hash energy and a hot egg moment. 70

Eggs in a Hot Tub – Where bold eggs simmer in style. 60

Fire & Lime Affair – A Latin dance party... in a bowl. 90

Flavor Jacuzzi – Like a spa day… but for your taste buds. 82

Flat Out Fabulous – When your veggies wanna party on a flatbread. 42

Frittata Me Not – Egg-citement, Served Hot. 72

Fry Me to the Moon – Stir-fried, sauced up, and ready for takeoff. 106

Get Your Wrap Together – Fresh, fast, fridge-friendly, crunch-worthy. 52

Holy Frijole – Loud, proud, and fully loaded. 76

In a Pickle (and Loving It) – Fridge-raided salad with serious bite. 96

Lemony Snickerdish – When life gives you lemons… make dinner. 88

Let's Have a Pep Talk – Bold bites tucked into bell pepper bliss. 56

Mac My Day – For when you need cheese therapy, fast. 64

Pasta La Vista, Boring – Because boring pasta deserves a swift exit. 100

Pastably Perfect Mini Bake – Bubbly, golden, and totally yours to devour. 48

Quesa Amor – Golden, gooey, and ready to wrap up your day. 104

Ricotta Be Kidding Me – Whipped, topped, and ready to toast your evening. 102

Shrimply Divine – Southern comfort meets solo sass in one buttery bowl. 50

Shroom for One – Creamy, dreamy, and just the fungi you need. 58

Soba Noodle Alla You – For rule-breakers who like their noodles with attitude. 86

Tabbouleh, Your Way – Herby, zesty, and totally fridge-freestyle. 94

Taco Me Later – Crunchy, punchy, and ready to party. 54

Tossed and Sauced – Sizzled, smothered, and straight-up seductive. 84

Umami in a Hurry – All aboard the flavor train (next stop: delicious). 74

Veggies Gone Wild – When the sheet pan turns into a flavor rave. 68

Wrap Me Baby One More Time – Hot, stuffed, and begging for seconds. 78

The Menu: Served by Style

Your flavor adventure, sorted by craving

Bake Squad

Bake It Till You Make It – Roasty, toasty, and smugly delicious. 66

Balls of Glory – Juicy little flavor bombs with veggie backup. 44

Let's Have a Pep Talk – Bold bites tucked into bell pepper bliss. 56

Egg-citing Eats

Egg-cellent for One – A solo frittata adventure—easy, breezy, and egg-stra tasty. 46

Egg-cuse Me, Dinner? – Bold hash energy and a hot egg moment. 70

Eggs in a Hot Tub – Where bold eggs simmer in style. 60

Frittata Me Not – Egg-citement, Served Hot. 72

Fresh Fix

In a Pickle (and Loving It) – Fridge-raided salad with serious bite. 96

Tabbouleh, Your Way – Herby, zesty, and totally fridge-freestyle. 94

Grainfully Delicious

Bowl'd & Boujee – Superfood star treatment, à la carte. 98

Holy Frijole – Loud, proud, and fully loaded. 76

Shrimply Divine – Southern comfort meets solo sass in one buttery bowl. 50

Taco Me Later – Crunchy, punchy, and ready to party. 54

Umami in a Hurry – All aboard the flavor train (next stop: delicious). 74

Veggies Gone Wild – When the sheet pan turns into a flavor rave. 68

Noodling Around

Mac My Day – For when you need cheese therapy, fast. 64

Pastably Perfect Mini Bake – Bubbly, golden, and totally yours to devour. 48

Pasta La Vista, Boring – Because boring pasta deserves a swift exit. 100

Tossed and Sauced – Sizzled, smothered, and straight-up seductive. 84

Slurp Worthy

Comfort in a Cup (or Bowl) – Sip, slurp, savor, repeat. 92

Curry Me Home – Creamy, cozy, and spoon-lickin' good. 40

Fire & Lime Affair – A Latin dance party... in a bowl. 90

Flavor Jacuzzi – Like a spa day… but for your taste buds. 82

Lemony Snickerdish – When life gives you lemons… make dinner. 88

Shroom for One – Creamy, dreamy, and just the fungi you need. 58

Snack-Cuterie

Board Out of My Mind – Dinner? Barely. Delicious? Absolutely. 108

Stir Crazy

Bangkok in a Pan – A flavor trip to Thailand, minus the jet lag. 62

Fry Me to the Moon – Stir-fried, sauced up, and ready for takeoff. 106

Soba Noodle Alla You – For rule-breakers who like their noodles with attitude. 86

Toastally Topped

Crust Me, It's Good – Golden, gooey, and gone in 60 seconds. 80

Flat Out Fabulous – When your veggies wanna party on a flatbread. 42

Queso Amor – Golden, gooey, and ready to wrap up your day. 104

Ricotta Be Kidding Me – Whipped, topped, and ready to toast your evening. 102

Wrap Stars

Get Your Wrap Together – Fresh, fast, fridge-friendly, crunch-worthy. 52

Wrap Me Baby One More Time – Hot, stuffed, and begging for seconds. 78

Bonus: Sauce It, Stir It, Drizzle It

One & Done Flavor Fun

Peanut Sauce, Please 114

Pesto Party for One 115

So Low Hummus 116

Sriracha Mayo (or Yogurt) 117

Chipotle Mayo (or Yogurt) 118

Quick Drizzles and Dollops

Avocado Crema 119

Yogurt-Tahini 119

Soy-Ginger Drizzle 119

Lime Vinaigrette 119

Simple Vinaigrette 119

About the Author

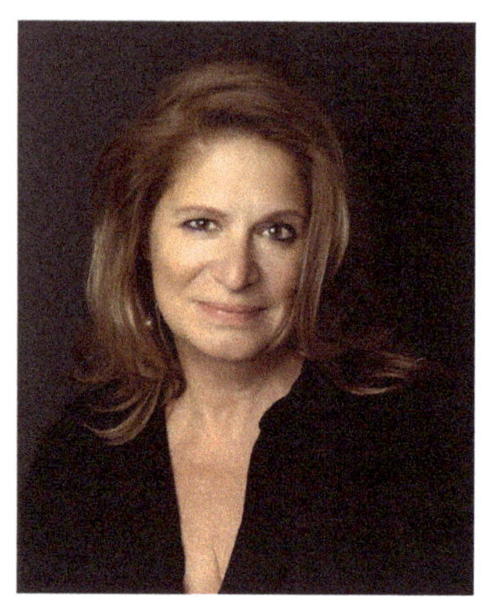

Kerstin Decook is a leadership coach, award-winning author, speaker, and unapologetic culinary enthusiast. She's the founder and flavor mentor behind Rock the Kitchen, where she helps home cooks ditch recipe fear, embrace flavor freedom, and actually have fun in the kitchen — one bold bite at a time.

But cooking wasn't always her thing.

Her path has been anything but ordinary — from a childhood behind the Iron Curtain in Russian-occupied East Germany to charting a life of adventure as a social educator, real estate agent, team manager, property wrangler, leadership coach, and eventually First Mate and Chef de Cuisine aboard the charter yacht she and her husband ran in the dreamy San Juan Islands.

It was during those yacht adventures that Kerstin realized... spaghetti and meatballs weren't gonna cut it. So she trained in culinary arts across the U.S., Canada, and Europe, diving deep into the *why* of good food — not just the how.

Now, she's on a mission to help thousands of home cooks feel proud, creative, and completely in control of what they serve.

Through her workshops, books, and a kitchen bubbling with love, laughter, and a whole lotta flavor, Kerstin helps women — and the bold men who dare — cook up a life that's as delicious as it is fulfilling.

Check out more at **RockTheKitchen.net** and **BreakLooseAndFly.com**

www.ingramcontent.com/pod-product-compliance
Ingram Content Group UK Ltd.
Pitfield, Milton Keynes, MK11 3LW, UK
UKHW061952290726
14090UKWH00021B/1191